Allergies FOR DUMMIES®

POCKET EDITION

by William E. Berger, MD, MBA

Look for Pocket Editions on these other topics:

Anxiety & Depression For Dummies, Pocket Edition
Asthma For Dummies, Pocket Edition
Diabetes For Dummies, Pocket Edition
Dieting For Dummies, Pocket Edition
Heart Disease For Dummies, Pocket Edition
High Blood Pressure For Dummies, Pocket Edition
Menopause For Dummies, Pocket Edition
Migraines For Dummies, Pocket Edition

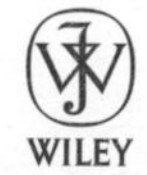

Wiley Publishing, Inc.

Allergies For Dummies®, Pocket Edition

Published by
Wiley Publishing, Inc.
111 River St.
Hoboken, NJ 07030-5774
www.wiley.com

For general information on our other products and services, please contact our Customer Care Department within the U.S. at 800-762-2974, outside the U.S. at 317-572-3993, or fax 317-572-4002.

For technical support, please visit www.wiley.com/techsupport.

Wiley also publishes its books in a variety of electronic formats. Some content that appears in print may not be available in electronic books.

Library of Congress Control Number: 2005936638

ISBN–13: 978-0-471-79232-1

ISBN–10: 0-471-79232-2

Manufactured in the United States of America

10 9 8 7 6 5 4 3 2 1

1O/TQ/RS/QV/IN

Publisher's Acknowledgments

Project Editor: Georgette Beatty
Copy Editor: Melissa Wiley
Composition Services: Indianapolis Composition Services Department
Cover Photo: © Getty Images/Stockbyte

Table of Contents

Introduction

How are you feeling? Do you or does someone you know think that having allergies means that feeling unwell is normal and that your condition can never improve? Unfortunately, many people answer "yes" to this question. However, as I explain throughout this book, the plain, simple, and accurate medical truth is this: Although no cure exists for allergies, when you receive effective, appropriate care from your doctor, combined with your motivated participation as a patient, you can lead a normal, active, and fulfilling life.

About This Book

I wrote this book to give you sound, up-to-date, practical advice, based on my 25-plus years of experience with numerous patients, about dealing with your condition effectively and appropriately. For that reason, I structure this book so that you can jump to the sections that most directly apply to you. You don't need to read this book from cover to cover, although I won't object if you do.

This book can also serve as a reference and source for information about the many facets of diagnosing, treating, and managing your condition. Although you may pick up this book for one topic, you may realize later that other topics also apply to you or a loved one.

Don't worry about remembering where related subjects are in this book. I provide ample cross-references in every chapter that remind you where to look for the information you may need in other chapters or within other sections of the chapter that you're reading.

I intend the information in this book to help you to

- Set goals for your treatment
- Ensure that you receive the most appropriate and effective medical care
- Do your part as a patient by adhering to the treatment plan that you and your physician develop

Foolish Assumptions

I don't think I'm being too foolish, but I assume that you want substantive, scientifically accurate, relevant information about allergies, presented in everyday language, without a lot of medical mumbo jumbo. In this book, I provide straightforward explanations of important scientific information and key medical terms. (You also get a chance to work on your Latin and Greek.)

If you've chosen to read my book, I know you're no dummy, so I'm willing to go out on a limb and make some further assumptions about you, dear reader:

- You or someone you care about suffers from allergies.
- You want to educate yourself about allergies as part of improving your medical condition (in consultation with your doctor, of course).
- You want to feel better.
- You really like doctors named Bill.

Icons Used in This Book

Throughout the margins of the book, you may notice the following icons. They're intended to catch your attention and alert you to the type of information I present in particular paragraphs. Here's what they mean:

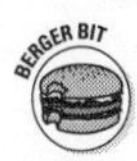

The Berger Bit icon represents me expressing my opinion.

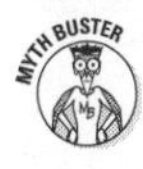

Myths and misconceptions abound about allergies. The Myth Buster icon indicates where I expose and correct mistaken beliefs that many people hold about allergies.

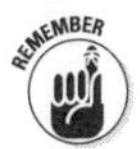

The Remember icon indicates things you shouldn't forget because you may find the information useful in the future.

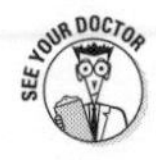

The See Your Doctor icon alerts you to matters that you should discuss with your physician.

To give you as complete a picture as possible, I occasionally get into more complex details of medical science. The Technical Stuff icon lets you know that's what I'm doing so that you can delve into the topic further — or skip it. You don't have to read these paragraphs to understand the subject at hand. (However, reading the information with these icons may give you a better handle on managing your medical condition.)

You can find plenty of helpful information and advice in paragraphs marked with the Tip icon.

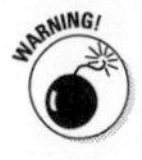

A Warning icon advises you about potential problems, such as symptoms you shouldn't ignore or treatments that you may not want to undergo.

Where to Go from Here

Although you can read this book from cover to cover if you want, I suggest turning to the Table of Contents and finding the sections that apply to your immediate concern. Then begin reading your way to better management of your condition.

If you want even more information on allergies and asthma, from the basic facts to managing allergies and asthma, check out the full-size version of *Asthma For Dummies* — simply head to your local book seller or go to `www.dummies.com`!

Chapter 1

Hay Fever 101

In This Chapter

- Appreciating appropriate hay fever management
- Differentiating among various forms of hay fever
- Keeping an eye on the triggers
- Seeking a doctor's opinion and treatment
- Managing hay fever

Hay fever (known medically as *allergic rhinitis*) is the most common allergic disease in the United States and often coexists with asthma. As many as 45 million Americans may suffer from some form of hay fever, including 10 to 30 percent of all adults and up to 40 percent of all children. That's a lot of sneezing fits, runny noses, clogged sinuses, and itchy, watery eyes.

Hay fever affects so many people that the estimated costs of medical treatment, absenteeism, and lost productivity from this type of allergy are perhaps as high as $11 billion annually in the United States. U.S. school children with hay fever miss the equivalent of 1.5 million school days per year and are at an increased risk of

- Experiencing developmental delays (such as hearing and speech difficulties)
- Suffering from poor school performance (due to drowsiness and irritability)

- Developing learning disabilities (due to poor focus and concentration)
- Having emotional and behavioral problems

Although the effects of hay fever are rarely life-threatening (though some people sometimes feel as if they could die when symptoms take hold), hay fever can still be a debilitating disease with serious consequences if you don't treat and manage it appropriately — especially if you have asthma. That's because the allergic reactions associated with hay fever are among the most serious and frequent triggers of respiratory symptoms in the vast majority of asthma patients.

Your respiratory tract is what I like to call the *united airway,* and treating your nose is often essential in treating the underlying inflammation that characterizes asthma.

Catching Up with Your Runny Nose

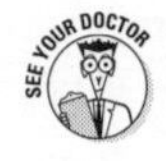

Although often called hay fever, allergic rhinitis itself doesn't cause fever. If you do run a temperature while experiencing symptoms that resemble hay fever, you may actually be suffering from a viral or bacterial infection, such as sinusitis, influenza (flu), or pneumonia.

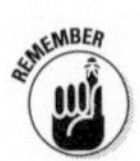

To effectively and appropriately manage your hay fever, I strongly advise you to consider the following factors:

- **You're in it for the long-term:** This disease usually recurs persistently and indefinitely after you've become sensitized to the allergens that trigger hay fever symptoms.

- **You need a healthy nose:** Because your nose is such a vital part of your respiratory system, your nasal health is vital to your overall wellness. Lack of treatment or ineffective or inappropriate management of hay fever can lead to complications such as nasal polyps (outgrowths of the nasal lining), sinusitis (inflammation of the sinuses; see Chapter 5), recurrent ear infections (potentially causing hearing loss; see Chapter 5), aggravation of bronchial symptoms, dental and facial abnormalities, poor speech development in children, and disruption of normal sleep patterns, resulting in daytime fatigue.

  Not only does your nose hold up your sunglasses, but it also provides other beneficial functions. For instance, your nose helps to warm and humidify the air you breathe. Also, the interior of your nose acts to filter and cleanse the air you breathe in through the action of the *cilia* (tiny hairlike projections of certain types of cells that sweep mucus through the nose).

  Last but certainly not least, your nose is critical for your sense of smell and the quality of your voice. For example, when your nose is stuffy or congested, your voice often sounds different (often referred to as *nasal voice*).

- **You need to know why you're blowing your nose:** A proper diagnosis of your hay fever condition requires a review of your medical history, a physical examination, observation, analysis, and, in some cases, skin testing to identify the allergens involved, all to help determine the most effective course of treatment.

- **You need to avoid allergic triggers:** In many cases, the most effective and least expensive method of managing your hay fever is to avoid the allergens that trigger your symptoms. Although you may not be able to completely avoid all the allergens that cause your symptoms, partial avoidance may provide you with enough relief to substantially improve your quality of life.

- **You should be cautious when using medications:** If you suffer from hay fever, you may resort to common first-generation, over-the-counter (OTC) antihistamines, decongestants, and nasal sprays to relieve your symptoms. However, many of these medications often produce significant side effects, including drowsiness (seriously limiting the safe use of these antihistamines), impaired vision, hypertension, nausea, gastric distress, constipation, insomnia, and irritability — and that's the short list. Besides creating more havoc in your life than allergic rhinitis already provides, these side effects can also be potentially dangerous. Overusing OTC decongestant nasal sprays can also lead to a condition known as *nasal rebound.* See Chapter 3 for more on nasal rebound.
- **Your doctor can prescribe new and improved medication:** In cases where avoidance doesn't provide you with sufficient relief, newer and safer prescription drugs — including second-generation nonsedating and less-sedating antihistamines and nasal sprays — are often effective and produce fewer side effects than their OTC counterparts. However, these prescription drugs are effective only if you follow your doctor's instructions and take them properly.

Classifying Types of Hay Fever

Hay fever is a common and nonspecific term for many varied types of allergic rhinitis, and it's often used in a general manner when discussing nasal inflammatory disorders, as well as for selling hay fever medications.

Because the term *hay fever* describes so many different nasal inflammatory disorders, you may not be aware that allergists make distinctions between the different forms of allergic rhinitis. Allergists group these forms according to the various types and patterns of exposure.

The three principal classifications of hay fever are seasonal allergic rhinitis; perennial allergic rhinitis, including perennial allergic rhinitis with seasonal *exacerbation* (worsening); and occupational allergic rhinitis.

Seasonal allergic rhinitis

Seasonal allergic rhinitis is the most common form of allergic rhinitis, with symptoms occurring at specific times of the year when particular pollen or mold spore allergens are in the air.

Hay fever symptoms can vary from year to year, however, due to climatic conditions and regional differences that affect the quality and quantity of pollen and mold spores in the environment. Hay fever symptoms can also vary because of the timing and types of exposure that you experience to these substances.

The levels of wind-borne tree, grass, and weed pollens are usually at their peak in the United States and Canada during the following times of year:

- **Late winter (warmer climates) to late spring:** Tree pollens.
- **Late spring to early summer:** Grass pollens.
- **Midsummer to fall:** Weed pollens, especially ragweed, which accounts for up to three-quarters of seasonal allergic rhinitis cases in the United States. The presence of weed pollen may continue in warmer climates through December in the absence of an early frost.

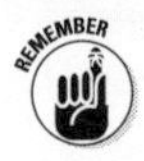

Wind-borne mold spores are present at various levels for most of the year, but they tend to cause a significant problem mostly during the late summer and fall.

Perennial allergic rhinitis

Perennial allergic rhinitis is usually the result of your immune system becoming sensitized to a triggering agent or combination of agents that are constantly present in the environment, whether in the home, outdoors, at work or school, or other locations that you frequent. The symptoms involved in this condition can be just as severe as the symptoms of seasonal allergic rhinitis.

During allergy or ragweed season, or at other times of the year when significant quantities of allergenic material are present, if you already have perennial allergic rhinitis, you may also experience a seasonal worsening of your allergies, resulting in even more disabling symptoms. Doctors refer to this condition as *perennial allergic rhinitis with seasonal exacerbation* (worsening).

In some cases, consistent and long-term exposure to multiple allergens can also lead to *chronic allergic rhinitis,* which means that your allergy symptoms are severe on a constant basis.

Occupational allergic rhinitis

Occupational allergic rhinitis is more difficult to diagnose and treat than other forms of hay fever because it often involves various combinations of a multitude of potential triggering agents and irritants found in many workplaces and occupations. Also, this specific type of hay fever often affects people with occupational asthma.

Your doctor should determine the following factors in the course of diagnosing occupational allergic rhinitis:

- Do your symptoms primarily occur at work? Or, if already present elsewhere, do your symptoms worsen while in the workplace?
- Do your symptoms disappear or improve after you leave work — at the end of the day, during weekends or vacations, when your work location changes, or if you take a new job?
- Do any of your colleagues and coworkers experience similar allergic symptoms?

What Makes Noses Run?

In addition to wind-borne grass, weed, and tree pollens and mold spores, other allergic and nonallergic rhinitis triggers found in indoor environments include

- Dust mite allergens
- Indoor mold growths
- Animal dander, saliva, and urine from warm-blooded pets, such as dogs and cats
- Waste and remains of pests, such as mice, rats, and cockroaches
- Allergens found in workplaces, schools, or other indoor or enclosed locations that you frequent
- Allergenic substances such as fibers, latex, wood dust, various chemicals, and many other items

Many substances that don't trigger an allergic response from your body's immune system can still intensify allergy or asthma conditions. Allergists refer to these substances as *irritants.* Common types of irritants include tobacco smoke, aerosols, glue, household cleaners, perfumes and scents, and strongly scented soaps.

In some cases, changes in weather conditions can trigger symptoms of rhinitis in susceptible individuals.

Getting a Medical Evaluation

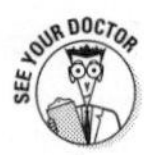

I strongly advise anyone who experiences significant hay fever symptoms — especially if you have asthma — to consult a physician to determine whether those symptoms are the result of a form of allergic rhinitis, a nonallergic type of rhinitis, a sinus infection, or a respiratory disease. A proper diagnosis is critical for the effective and appropriate management of any of these conditions.

Understanding that sneezy, itchy, and runny feeling

Many allergic rhinitis sufferers mistakenly assume that they have lingering colds that afflict them every spring (or whenever the weather changes). However, even though viral infections such as the common cold and flu may follow cyclical patterns, the frequency of these illnesses usually isn't as consistent or as constant as seasonal, perennial, or occupational allergic rhinitis.

Symptoms associated with these forms of allergic rhinitis may often include

- Runny nose with clear, watery discharge
- Nasal congestion (stuffy nose)

- Sneezing
- Postnasal drip (nasal discharge down the back of your throat)
- Itchy, watery eyes (allergic conjunctivitis)
- Itchy nose, ears, and throat
- Persistent irritation of the mucous membranes of the eyes, middle ear, nose, and sinuses (in chronic cases)

Approximately half of all patients with allergic rhinitis experience additional clinical symptoms due to a *late-phase reaction* occurring three to ten hours after allergen exposure, which typically leads to persistent symptoms, especially nasal congestion. The late-phase reaction is also implicated in *nonspecific reactivity* (increased sensitivity) of the nasal lining to nonallergic irritants.

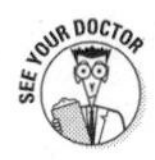

Allergic rhinitis usually does *not* cause symptoms such as fever, sore throat, green or yellow thickened nasal drainage, achy muscles or joints, or tooth or eye pain. If you're experiencing these types of symptoms, the source of your ailment may be a type of viral or bacterial infection or the result of some physical factor, such as an injury. Your doctor should evaluate your condition.

If you have a deviated (crooked) septum (the *septum* is the bony cartilage between your nostrils), it can block one or both sides of your nose, leading to a runny or congested nose. Because the resulting symptoms resemble allergic rhinitis, examination of your septum should be part of your physical examination. Surgical correction of a deviated septum may be necessary to relieve severe nasal airway obstruction.

Telltale signs: Salutes, shiners, and creases

The symptoms of allergic rhinitis that I list in this chapter often produce a distinctive combination of gestures and facial features, particularly in children and adolescents. If you or someone close to you seems to suffer from allergic rhinitis, keep the following sufferer-specific characteristics in mind. The physical signs of allergic rhinitis are often so unique that I can usually tell when looking in the waiting room who the likely allergic rhinitis sufferers are. When my children were younger, I noticed similar traits among their friends who had allergies as well.

The following gestures and facial formations are characteristics that you and your doctor should look for to help diagnose your specific condition:

- **Allergic salute:** As tempting as it may be to consider this gesture a sign of respect for your doctor, the allergic salute actually describes the way that most people use the palm of their hand to rub and raise the tip of their nose to relieve nasal itching and congestion (and possibly to wipe away some mucus).
- **Allergic shiner:** Allergic rhinitis symptoms can really beat up some patients. Dark circles under the eyes, due to the swelling and discoloration caused by congestion of small blood vessels beneath the skin in this area, can give you the appearance of having gone a few rounds in a boxing match.
- **Allergic (adenoidal) face:** Allergic rhinitis may cause swelling of the *adenoids* (lymph tissue that lines the back of the throat and extends behind the nose), resulting in a sort of tired and droopy appearance.
- **Nasal crease:** This line across the bridge of the nose is usually the result — particularly in children — of

rubbing the nose (allergic salute) to relieve nasal congestion and itching.

- **Mouth breathing:** Cases of allergic rhinitis in which severe nasal congestion occurs can result in chronic mouth breathing, leading to the development of a high, arched palate, an elevated upper lip, and an overbite. (This symptom is one of the main reasons why so many teens with allergic rhinitis wind up at the orthodontist.)

Seeing red: Allergic conjunctivitis

Symptoms such as redness over your eyeballs and the underside of your eyelids, as well as swollen, itchy, and tearing eyes, are characteristic of what doctors refer to as *allergic conjunctivitis.* This ailment often coexists with allergic rhinitis, and most of the same allergens as those involved with allergic rhinitis can trigger seasonal or perennial outbreaks of this conjunctivitis.

All that drips isn't allergic

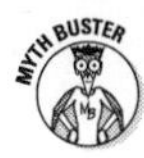

Many people think that runny, congested noses and sneezing are always the result of an allergic reaction. However, be aware that rhinitis also comes in nonallergic flavors, such as the following types:

- **Infectious:** Upper respiratory viral ailments such as the common cold are often the cause of acute or chronic nasal distress.
- **Hormonal:** Women may experience severe nasal congestion while taking birth control pills, as well as during ovulation or pregnancy — most notably from the second month to the full term. In pregnancy cases, congested nose symptoms usually disappear after delivery.

- **Emotional:** Women and men may experience runny and congested noses during sexual arousal. Other intense emotional reactions (such as laughing or crying) can also provoke your nose to run or congest.
- **Vasomotor:** The most typical examples of this form of nonallergic rhinitis are the nasal congestion, runny nose, and sneezing that can occur as a result of sudden weather or temperature changes (for example, a blast of cold air). Exposure to bright lights or irritants, such as tobacco smoke, perfume, bleach, paint fumes, newsprint, automotive emissions, and solvents, can also trigger vasomotor rhinitis.
- **Drug-induced:** Anti-hypertensives (medications for high blood pressure), as well as aspirin and nonsteroidal anti-inflammatory drugs (NSAIDs) like ibuprofen, can also induce symptoms of a runny or congested nose. Overusing OTC nasal decongestant sprays (Afrin, Neo-Synephrine) can lead to chronic drug-induced nasal congestion (due to nasal rebound from the medication), a condition that doctors describe as *rhinitis medicamentosa.*

  Abused illegal drugs, such as cocaine, can also produce rhinitis symptoms.
- **Gustatory:** Hot, spicy foods — especially those with serious peppers — can provoke watery eyes, runny noses, and sneezing (and temporarily clear sinuses in the process — whew!). Beer, wine, and other types of alcoholic drinks can also produce these sorts of symptoms in some people.

  This type of immediate, localized nonallergic reaction to certain types of cuisine and alcoholic beverages isn't the same as the more complex allergic process that occurs with a food allergy, as I explain in Chapter 6.

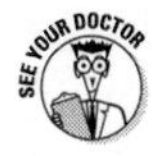

To effectively diagnose your condition, a physician must review your medical history, as well as your family's history of allergies, and perform a physical examination. If your family doctor suspects a form of allergic rhinitis, he will probably refer you to a specialist, such as an allergist (someone like me) or an otolaryngologist (an ear, nose, and throat doctor), in the following situations:

- If clarification and identification of the triggers of your condition are needed
- If the management of your allergic or nonallergic rhinitis isn't resulting in a substantial improvement of your condition due to inadequate treatment or adverse reactions to medications
- If you need to find out how to avoid allergens and irritants that may be triggering your symptoms
- If your rhinitis or side effects of medications for the condition impair your abilities to perform in your career or occupation (especially in operating an airplane or motor vehicle)
- If the disease has a significant adverse effect on your quality of life by affecting your comfort and well-being
- If rhinitis complications develop, such as sinusitis, *otitis* (ear inflammation), and facial signs (see the "Telltale signs: Salutes, shiners, and creases" sidebar, earlier in this chapter)
- If you have coexisting conditions, such as recurring or chronic sinusitis (see Chapter 5), asthma or another respiratory condition, otitis (see Chapter 5), or nasal polyps
- If your doctor needs to prescribe oral (systemic) corticosteroids (see Chapter 4) to control your symptoms

- If your symptoms last more than three months
- If your medication costs are a financial hardship

Knowing what the doctor's looking for

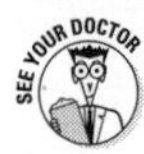

In addition to performing a general observation to check for the hallmarks of allergic rhinitis (see the sidebar "Telltale signs: Salutes, shiners, and creases," earlier in this chapter), your doctor will most likely examine the following areas:

- The front of your nose, to check for an allergic crease and the condition of your *septum* (the "great divide" of cartilage between your nostrils).
- Your nasal passages, to check for swelling of the nasal *turbinates* (protruding tissues that line the interior of the nose — see Figure 1-1); nasal *polyps* (pale, round or pear-shaped, smooth, gelatinous outgrowths of the nasal lining); congestion; and the character, color, and amount of secretions from your nose.
- The inside of your mouth and the back of your throat, to check for redness, swelling, enlarged or diseased tonsils and to check drainage from the nasal cavity. In addition, your doctor may check for the presence of a high, arched palate and *malocclusion* (misalignment of the jaw and teeth due to mouth breathing and tongue thrusting).
- Your neck and face, to check for lumps and sensitive, painful, or numb areas.
- Your eyes and ears, to check for signs of inflammation and infection.
- If indicated, further examination may include checking your vocal cords, adenoids, sinuses, and *Eustachian tubes* (the connection between your middle ear, nose, and throat that causes your ears to pop when descending in an airplane).

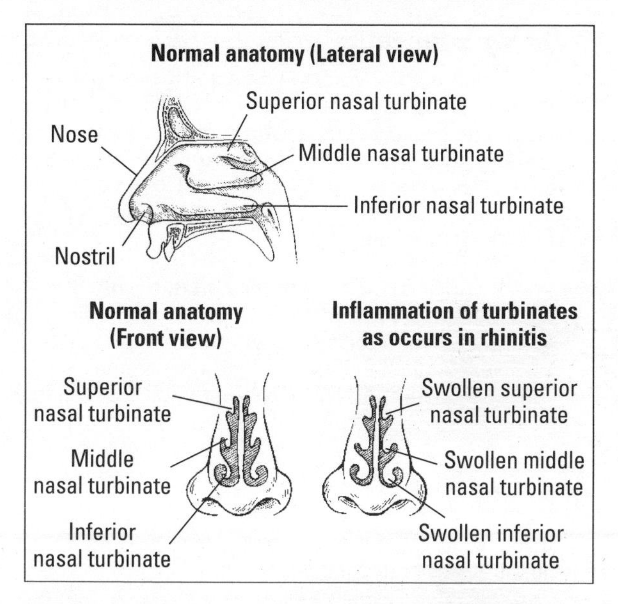

Figure 1-1: The two cross sections show the difference between a healthy nose and one with rhinitis.

In addition to evaluating your physiological condition, your physician also attempts to determine

- The pattern, frequency, and seasonal variations of the allergic reactions that you experience.
- The types of allergens and irritants to which you may be exposed at home, work, school, friends' and relatives' homes, and other locations that you frequent, such as malls, theaters, restaurants, and even modes of transport, such as vehicles, trains, boats, and airplanes.

Doing your part

You can also keep track of when and where your allergic symptoms occur in order to help with the diagnostic process. For example, you may experience mild but manageable hay fever symptoms when visiting friends who have dogs and cats. However, you may find that, on occasion, your symptoms from those visits are more severe.

If you can track the times and dates of your allergic episodes, you can greatly help your doctor in determining whether the presence of seasonal allergens such as ragweed may worsen your condition by increasing your allergen load.

Managing Rhinitis

Three basic approaches exist for treating and managing allergies.

Avoiding allergens

Benjamin Franklin once advised, "An ounce of prevention is worth a pound of cure." Eliminating (or at least lessening) your exposure to allergens and irritants can often result in less severe symptoms and less need for medication.

Treating with medications

Pharmacotherapy is the term doctors use for treating patients with medications. This form of therapy is particularly important in allergic diseases, because complete avoidance of allergens can be difficult. Therefore, your doctor may also recommend or prescribe one or more medications to help manage your condition, depending on the nature and severity of your symptoms, occupation, age, and other factors that your physician may assess. I provide an in-depth analysis of these products and their recommended uses and side effects in Chapters 3 and 4.

Treating the cause of your allergies

If your doctor concludes that avoidance and drug therapies don't provide effective results, and if the severity of your symptoms or the nature of your occupation warrants it, your doctor may advise you to consider *immunotherapy,* otherwise known as *desensitization, hyposensitization,* or just plain-old *allergy shots.* Immunotherapy treatment for allergic rhinitis generally requires at least three years of injections. For an in-depth discussion of immunotherapy, turn to Chapter 2.

Considering special cases

Certain groups of hay fever patients require more specialized treatment and consideration:

- **Children:** Oral antihistamines and mast-cell stabilizer sprays (nasal cromolyn, such as Nasalcrom) are currently the first medication options for younger patients who experience allergic rhinitis symptoms. Your family doctor may also consider prescription nasal corticosteroid sprays (Flonase, Rhinocort AQ).
- **Elderly people:** Doctors generally advise that elderly patients use nonsedating antihistamines, which produce fewer significant side effects, instead of first-generation OTC antihistamine products (see Chapters 3 and 4 for details about allergic rhinitis medications).

In addition, nasal corticosteroids are often recommended for elderly patients. Doctors often warn patients (usually in the elderly age group) with insomnia, prostate problems, hypertension, and heart conditions to avoid taking oral decongestants, because the medications can possibly aggravate their preexisting medical problems.

- **Pregnant women:** Physicians often consider mast-cell stabilizer sprays (nasal cromolyn, such as Nasalcrom) as the first medication option for the relief of allergic rhinitis symptoms among pregnant women. During the first trimester of pregnancy, your doctor may advise you to avoid oral decongestants. However, after the first trimester of pregnancy, your doctor may recommend antihistamines such as chlorpheniramine (Chlor-Trimeton), loratadine (Claritin), and cetirizine (Zyrtec) or nasal corticosteroids such as budesonide (Rhinocort AQ).
- **Athletes:** Your doctor needs to make sure that any recommended or prescribed OTC or prescription product isn't on any sports federation's list of banned substances. The U.S. Olympic Committee (USOC) and the International Olympic Committee ban the use of all oral and nasal decongestants and oral corticosteroids. In addition, some international sports federations also ban the use of oral antihistamines. Using other nasal products may require written approval by governing sports bodies.

  Obviously, whether the use of a product is governed or not, if you're an athlete, you need to avoid any medication that may adversely affect your performance or give you an unfair competitive advantage.

Chapter 2

Getting Allergy Tested and Allergy Shots

In This Chapter

- Using your skin test results
- Making informed choices about immunotherapy

Depending on the severity and nature of your asthma and allergies (such as allergic rhinitis, or *hay fever*) and the degree of your exposure to allergens that trigger your respiratory symptoms, avoidance measures and *pharmacotherapy* (treatment with medications) may not be all that you require for effectively managing your condition. You may also need to identify and address root causes of your condition instead of simply treating your symptoms. As a result, your doctor may refer you to an allergist for skin tests and possible immunotherapy.

Doctors use skin tests to confirm that your symptoms result from allergies instead of some other cause. Doctors also use skin tests to identify, if possible, the specific allergens that trigger your allergic symptoms and reactions and asthma symptoms.

Meanwhile, *immunotherapy* is also known as *allergy shots, desensitization, hyposensitization,* or *allergy vaccination.* The advisability of this treatment depends on whether skin testing provides clear evidence that you're allergic to specific allergens, what those allergens are, and how they correlate with your medical history.

This chapter takes a closer look at both of these specialized diagnostic and treatment procedures so you know what to expect.

Diagnosing with Skin Tests

Allergists consider skin tests the most reliable and precise method for diagnosing allergies.

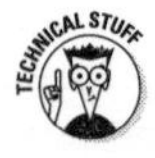

Doctors use skin tests to determine whether a minute dose of a suspected allergen — which an allergist or clinic staff member administers in solution form on or just below your skin — produces a small-scale, localized positive response known as a *wheal and erythema (flare) reaction.* A wheal and erythema reaction is a reddened and small-scale swelling of your skin that resembles a mosquito bite, hive, or bump at the site of the allergen test. A positive reaction confirms that you have sensitivity to the administered allergen but may also indicate your specific sensitivity level to that allergen.

After completion of the skin tests, you should remain under observation for at least 30 minutes. If the tests produce a positive reaction, your allergist or test administrator examines and measures the resulting wheal and erythema. Clinicians use these measurements to help determine your level of sensitivity to the specific allergen that was administered. If your physician concludes that you need immunotherapy, knowing your level of sensitivity to the allergen often is important in determining a safe starting dosage for your first series of allergy shots.

Pins and needles

Most allergists use two types of skin tests to evaluate allergic ailments:

- **Prick-puncture:** Sometimes referred to as a *scratch test,* clinicians perform this test on the surface of your back or on your forearm.
- **Intracutaneous:** Allergists perform this test, also known as *intradermal testing,* only when the prick-puncture test fails to produce a significant positive result. This test involves a series of small injections of allergen solution in rows just below the surface of the skin on your arm or forearm.

For both prick-puncture and intracutaneous tests, a positive reaction usually appears within 20 minutes. With either test, you needn't worry about someone turning you into a pincushion or sticking you with a giant syringe. The intracutaneous test uses only very fine needles just beneath the surface of the skin and, like the prick-puncture test (on the surface of the skin), produces minimal discomfort.

Skin tests and antihistamines: Not a good mix

After carefully reviewing your condition and history, if your doctor advises skin testing, you probably need to discontinue using your antihistamine medications (and other products in certain cases, but usually not your asthma drugs) for several days prior to the test. The presence of these drugs in your body can interfere with the skin-test results. However, it's unlikely that you'll need to stop most of your other medications.

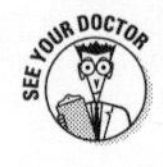

Never abruptly stop taking your asthma medications without first checking with your doctor. Fortunately, most asthma medications don't interfere with allergy skin testing.

The following list offers some general guidelines about discontinuing various common products; however, your allergist can provide you with more exact instructions based on the specific medications that you take.

- Discontinue older, sedating, first-generation, over-the-counter (OTC) antihistamines, such as Benadryl, Chlor-Trimeton, Dimetapp, Tavist-1, and similar products, for 48 to 72 hours before your skin test.
- You may need to stop using newer, nonsedating, second-generation antihistamines, such as Allegra, Clarinex (and its OTC precursor, Claritin), Zyrtec, or Seldane, for as long as two to four days prior to testing. Likewise, studies show that Hismanal can interfere when taken up to three months prior to having skin tests. Therefore, you and your physician need to plan accordingly whenever you take Hismanal and anticipate taking a skin test. (Seldane and Hismanal are no longer are available in the United States but still are sold in Canada and other countries; see Chapter 3.)
- Make sure your allergist knows if you're taking beta blockers (Inderal, Tenormin) or monoamine oxidase inhibitors (Nardil, Parnate), because special precautions must be taken when administering skin tests to patients who take these drugs. They sometimes can render epinephrine ineffective. *Epinephrine* is a rescue medication that doctors use for emergency treatment in cases when

rare, severe allergic reactions occur following skin testing.

- Because some of them have antihistamine effects, certain antidepressants also can interfere with skin tests. If you're taking antidepressants, such as trycyclic antidepressants (Elavil or Sinequan), check with the doctor who prescribed them to find out whether you can safely stop taking those products for a brief period or whether substituting another antidepressant (such as Prozac or Paxil) that doesn't have antihistaminic properties is possible. If discontinuing these drugs to undergo skin testing is permitted, you may need to stop taking them for three to five days prior to your test. Don't ever stop taking any prescribed medication (for any medical condition) without first checking with your doctor.
- Skin conditions such as contact dermatitis, eczema, psoriasis, or lesions (irritations) in the skin-test area also can interfere with your test results. Make sure that your doctor knows about any such conditions before you undergo any skin testing.

Prick-puncture procedures

Allergists consider prick-puncture tests the most convenient and cost-effective screening method for detecting *specific IgE antibodies,* which are produced by your immune system in response to a wide variety of inhalant and food allergens.

When performing a prick-puncture test, an allergist or other qualified medical professional first places a drop of a suspected allergen (in solution form) on your back or forearm. The test administrator then uses a device that pricks, punctures, or scratches the area to see whether the allergen produces a reaction. The device merely scrapes the skin, without drawing blood.

Alternatively, multiple prick-puncture tests can be administered simultaneously with a *Multi-Test* — a sterile, disposable multiple skin-test applicator with eight heads. This procedure uses an applicator that has a specific allergen extract on each of its eight applicator heads and is applied directly to the patient's skin, as shown in Figure 2-1.

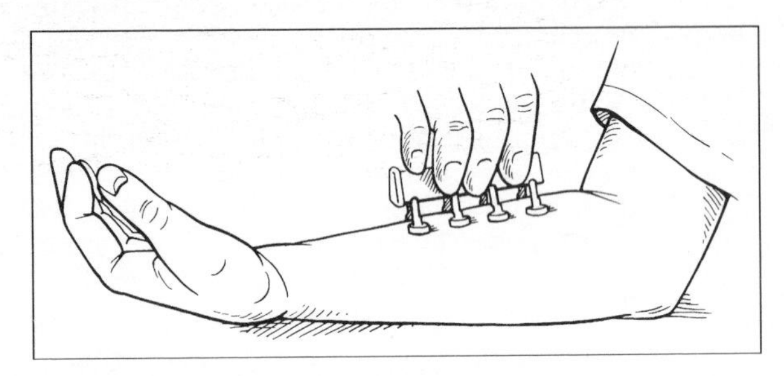

Figure 2-1: A multiple skin-test applicator can be used to administer prick-puncture skin tests.

You may have to undergo as many as 70 prick-puncture tests to conclusively identify inhalant allergens. The number of tests you receive varies according to factors such as the area where you live, work, or go to school and the types of allergen exposure that you receive. In many cases, your doctor requires fewer tests.

The number of prick-puncture tests that your doctor may need to administer to determine your specific food allergies varies from 20 to 80. However, only a few selected foods (milk, eggs, peanuts, tree nuts, fish, shellfish, soy, and wheat) account for the vast majority of cases of allergic food reactions. By first taking a detailed medical history, in many cases your doctor may need to perform only a few carefully chosen food-allergen skin tests to confirm a likely diagnosis of *food hypersensitivity,* or food allergy (see Chapter 6).

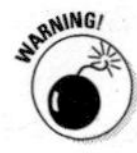

Some food allergies, such as peanut hypersensitivity, can trigger serious reactions. Whenever a patient tells me, "Doctor, anytime I eat anything that has peanuts in it, I nearly die," I take his or her word for it. If you suffer from specific, severe food allergy reactions, I strongly advise against skin tests — and never recommend intracutaneous tests — because the resulting positive reaction can produce serious or even life-threatening results. Before you have any skin test, always tell your doctor about any serious food reactions that you may have experienced.

Intracutaneous testing

If your prick-puncture tests are inconclusive, your doctor may need to perform up to 40 intracutaneous tests — rarely that many in the case of suspected food allergies — to produce a significant positive reaction and confirm the diagnosis of an allergy.

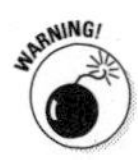

Because intracutaneous tests involve injecting an allergen extract just below the surface of your skin, the risk — although small — of a widespread systemic reaction exists. Rarely should an intracutaneous test be done for a particular allergen without a prior prick-puncture test for that same allergen. The type of adverse reaction that can result from administering a particular allergen usually is far less serious with a prick-puncture test, and it alerts your allergist to the potential danger of performing an intracutaneous test with that allergen.

Because of a variety of factors, including the types of allergen extracts that your allergist administers, delayed reactions can occur with prick-puncture tests but occur more often following intracutaneous tests. The characteristic signs of these reactions include swollen, reddened, numb bumps at the skin-test site.

Delayed reactions can develop 3 to 10 hours after your test and may continue for up to 12 hours thereafter. The bumps usually disappear 24 to 48 hours later. These delayed reactions, known as *late-phase skin reactions,* aren't a sign of immediate hypersensitivity, and allergists often tell their patients to ignore these late reactions.

Skin test side effects

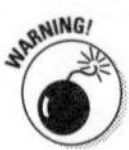

Skin testing occasionally produces adverse side effects in ultrasensitive individuals, but only rarely. As you'd expect, adverse reactions occur far less frequently with prick-puncture tests than with more invasive intracutaneous tests. These side effects can range from large local reactions on the skin to systemic reactions, such as sneezing, coughing, tightness of the chest, swelling of the throat, itchy eyes, and postnasal drip.

In very rare cases, death from *anaphylaxis,* a life-threatening reaction that affects many organs simultaneously, has occurred following a skin test. For that reason, medical facilities where doctors perform skin tests need to have appropriate emergency equipment and drugs on hand in the unlikely event that using these items becomes necessary.

Blood testing for allergies

Although most allergists consider skin tests the gold standard for diagnosing allergies, they may not work for every patient. Your allergist may advise diagnosing your allergic condition with a blood test known as *radioallergensorbent testing* (RAST) or Enzyme-Linked Immunosorbent Assay (ELISA). Your doctor may advise you to have a blood test rather than a skin test for the following reasons:

- Your prescribing physician advises you not to discontinue medications such as antihistamines and antidepressants that can interfere with skin-test results.
- You suffer from a severe skin condition, such as widespread eczema or psoriasis (over a large part of your body), and your doctor is unable to find a suitable skin site for testing.
- Your sensitivity level to suspected allergens is so high that any administration of those allergens may result in potentially serious side effects (for example, a history of life-threatening reactions to the ingestion of peanuts). If this is the case, then avoid allergy skin testing.
- Problematic behavioral, physical, or mental conditions prevent you from cooperating with the skin-testing process.

Because RAST can require only one blood sample to analyze many allergens, this method may seem more convenient than skin testing. However, other than the exceptions I list earlier in this section, most allergists rarely use RAST because it isn't as accurate as skin testing and can result in an incomplete profile of your allergies. In addition, RAST is more expensive and time consuming, because a laboratory must analyze blood samples and report test results, which often takes at least two days. If your results return inconclusive, your allergist must perform the test again and wait for new results. In comparison, skin testing usually provides results on the spot, within 15 to 30 minutes.

Reviewing Immunotherapy

Immunotherapy (also known as *allergy shots, desensitization, hyposensitization,* or *allergy vaccination*) currently is the most effective form of treating the underlying immunologic mechanism that causes allergic conditions such as allergic rhinitis, allergic conjunctivitis, allergic asthma, and allergies to insect stings. However, immunotherapy at present doesn't provide a safe and effective treatment for food allergies.

Seeing how immunotherapy works

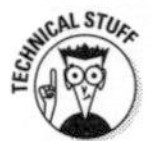

How exactly does immunotherapy work? The following info may help you understand it better:

- **Decreasing the production of IgE antibodies.** IgE antibodies are the agents that bind with allergens at receptor sites on the surfaces of mast cells, thus initiating the release of potent chemical mediators of inflammation, such as histamine and leukotrienes. These chemicals trigger allergic reactions and asthma symptoms.
- **Initiating the production of other allergen-specific IgG antibodies.** *Allergen-specific IgG antibodies* also are known as *blocking antibodies.* Immunotherapy can stimulate your body to produce blocking antibodies, which compete with mast-cell bound IgE for antigen, thus preventing the initial sensitization, activation, and subsequent release of potent chemical mediators of inflammation from these cells.
- **Stabilizing the actual mast cells (and basophils).** Doing so means that even if IgE antibodies and allergens cross-link on the surface of these cells, your potential allergic reaction is usually less severe because the release of potent chemical mediators of inflammation is reduced. In addition, immunotherapy can result in decreasing the actual number of mast cells (and basophils) in the affected areas. This reduction in activation and numbers of these cells also results in suppressing the inflammatory late-phase allergic response following allergen exposure.

Deciding whether immunotherapy makes sense for you

Immunotherapy may be appropriate for treating your allergies and thus can help you manage your asthma more effectively, depending on the following factors:

- Effectively avoiding allergens that trigger your allergic reactions and asthma symptoms is impractical, or even impossible, because the life you lead inevitably results in allergen exposure.
- Your respiratory symptoms are consistently severe or debilitating.
- Managing your allergies and/or asthma requires prohibitively expensive courses of medication, which produce side effects that adversely affect your overall health and quality of life. If the health and financial costs of multiple allergy drugs outweigh their benefits, immunotherapy may make more sense for you.
- Allergy testing provides conclusive evidence of specific IgE antibodies, thus enabling your allergist to identify the particular allergens that trigger your symptoms.
- You haven't experienced serious adverse side effects (as a result of skin testing) to the allergens that your doctor will use in your subsequent course of immunotherapy.
- You can make the commitment to see the therapy process through. Immunotherapy isn't a quick fix; it requires a significant investment of your time.

If you suffer from an unstable heart condition and you take beta blockers such as Inderal, if you have high blood pressure and take angiotensin-converting enzyme (ACE) inhibitors (Capoten, Vasotec), or if you take monoamine oxidase

(MAO) inhibitors (Nardil, Parnate), don't consider immunotherapy unless your physician advises you that the benefits of starting immunotherapy outweigh the risks of discontinuing those medications.

Getting shots

Injections, or shots, are the most effective and reliable method of administering specially prepared, diluted allergen extracts that allergists use when providing immunotherapy treatment. If needles give you nightmares, relax. Allergy shots are much less painful or traumatic than the deep intramuscular shots often needed to effectively administer immunizations or certain medications (such as cortisone or penicillin). That's because doctors usually administer allergy shots with the same type of fine needle they use in intracutaneous testing, thus causing minimal discomfort.

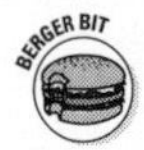

I'm often amazed at how well kids handle allergy shots after getting over their initial fears about that first shot. After the first shot, allergy shots aren't usually a problem for most children, especially when they notice that their respiratory symptoms are starting to improve. I don't claim that kids love getting allergy shots (or going to the doctor for anything besides a lollipop), but they usually quickly discover that receiving these injections beats not being able to breathe properly.

Allergens that doctors commonly use in immunotherapy treatments for allergic asthma, allergic rhinitis, and allergic conjunctivitis include extracts of inhalant allergens from tree, grass, and weed pollens; mold spores; dust mites; and sometimes animal danders.

In preparing your allergen extract (serum or vaccine), your doctor includes only those allergens for which you previously have demonstrated sensitivity in your skin testing. If your skin tests show sensitivity to multiple allergens (you're sensitive to many grass and weed pollens, for example), your allergist may mix all the different grass extracts into one vial and all the different weed extracts into another vial. Preparing the serum in such combinations ensures that you receive only one shot for each group of extracts, thus reducing the number of injections that you need for effective therapy.

Your allergist may even determine that mixing doses of all your allergens into a single shot on a particular visit is an option for you based on:

- Your allergic sensitivity
- The volume of extract that needs to be administered
- The types of allergen extracts your allergist uses for your therapy

In some cases, for your comfort, it may be preferable to split the required dose of your allergy shot into two or more separate injections.

Although this treatment can greatly reduce your allergy symptoms, immunotherapy isn't considered a guaranteed permanent cure for asthma and allergies. You likewise still need to continue practicing avoidance measures while receiving immunotherapy, because doing so can significantly enhance the effectiveness of your treatment.

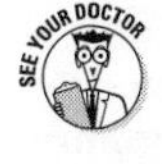

Immunotherapy can significantly improve your respiratory symptoms, thus reducing your need for allergy medication, which, in turn, makes this treatment the closest thing to a currently available cure for allergies and the respiratory symptoms they trigger. However, always tell your allergist:

- Whenever you're considering taking medications — including OTC drugs — for allergies or nonallergic conditions.
- About any changes in your medical condition, even if the changes may not seem directly connected to your allergies.
- Pregnancy, which I mention in the nearby sidebar, is an example of a change in medical condition that you need to report to your allergist.

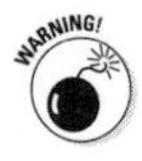

Your adherence is key for an effective immunotherapy program. Follow and maintain the shot schedule that your allergist prescribes as closely as possible. However, avoid shots under the following circumstances:

- **Exercise:** Make sure that you don't engage in strenuous physical activity for at least one hour before and two hours after your allergy shots. Exercising at these times can increase your risk of experiencing a serious adverse reaction, because exercise increases your blood circulation, potentially resulting in a rapid absorption of the allergen from the shot and possibly even causing a severe reaction.
- **Illness:** If you run a fever, tell your allergist. Receiving an allergy shot while you're ill isn't a good idea, because your fever symptoms can make detecting an adverse reaction to the shots difficult.
- **Immunizations:** Try to avoid scheduling any immunizations on the same day as your allergy shots; potential adverse effects from the immunization can make a reaction from an allergy

shot difficult to identify. If you get an immunization shot on the day of your scheduled allergy shots, let your allergist know; your allergist may advise you to not get your allergy shots that same day.

The most effective way of administering immunotherapy is by providing *perennial therapy,* which involves receiving shots of allergen extracts year-round. Studies show that perennial therapy provides the longest and most successful reduction of your level of sensitivity to specific allergens.

A typical course of perennial immunotherapy may follow these steps:

1. **Your allergist begins your therapy by administering shots once or twice a week, starting with a very small amount of a diluted dose of allergen extracts.**
2. **Your allergist gradually increases your allergen dosage by increasing the amount and concentration of the extract week by week until you reach the maintenance dose in about three to six months.** The *maintenance dose* refers to a predetermined amount of maximal concentration, or the highest strength that you can tolerate without producing adverse reactions.
3. **After reaching your maintenance dose, allergy symptom relief usually begins. When relief starts, you can continue receiving shots at the maintenance dose level.** Likewise, your allergist may extend the interval between your shots from one week to as many as four, depending on your response to the treatment and the levels of exposure that you encounter in your environment.

Pregnancy and immunotherapy

If you become pregnant while receiving immunotherapy, you'll be glad to know that your allergy shots are safe during pregnancy. In fact, your allergist may advise you to continue receiving immunotherapy, possibly at a reduced dosage, to minimize any risk of reactions to allergy shots and to continue to provide relief from your respiratory symptoms.

If you stop treatment, you can run the risk of experiencing worsening symptoms. This worsening can lead in turn to increased needs for medication that may not be desirable during your pregnancy. However, if you're already pregnant and are considering whether to start a course of immunotherapy, your allergist may advise you to delay beginning this form of treatment until after delivery.

Every time you receive your allergy shots, expect to wait at least 20 minutes afterwards in your allergist's office so that a medical staff member can inspect and evaluate the areas of skin around your shots and monitor you for any early signs of anaphylaxis. Another benefit of staying in your allergist's office after your shot: In the rare event that you experience a severe reaction, qualified medical personnel can immediately provide emergency assistance.

For inhalant allergens, an effective immunotherapy program usually requires shots for at least three to five years. In many cases, if your sensitivity to allergens improves during the course of immunotherapy, you can maintain your level of allergy improvement for several years (or even life-long in some cases) after discontinuing the shots.

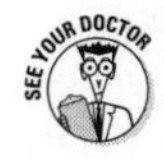

However, in some cases, withdrawing from immunotherapy results in the reappearance of allergic symptoms. Therefore, your allergist needs to evaluate the specifics of your individual case when considering the possibility of discontinuing immunotherapy.

Considering side effects

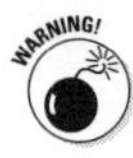

The possibility — however small — of anaphylactic reactions exists any time your allergist injects allergenic proteins into your body. In some unfortunate cases, people have died after receiving their allergy shots. Therefore, although the odds of a serious reaction to allergy shots are far less than those of getting into a bad car crash on the way to your allergist's office, take as many precautions as possible. After receiving an allergy shot, immediately tell your doctor or nurse if you're experiencing any of the following signs of serious adverse side effects:

- Itchiness of the feet, hands, groin area, and underarms
- Large-scale skin reactions, such as hives or flushing
- Upper and lower respiratory symptoms, such as sneezing, coughing, tightness of the chest, a swollen or itchy throat, itchy eyes, postnasal drip, difficulty swallowing, and a hoarse voice
- Nausea, diarrhea, and stomach cramps
- Dizziness, fainting, or a severe drop in blood pressure

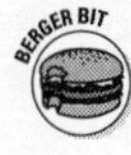

Because the threat of severe adverse reactions exists, I strongly advise against giving yourself allergy shots at home. Although practices vary in different areas, the vast majority of my colleagues insist that patients receive their allergy shots only in an appropriate medical facility, because of this small chance of adverse, life-threatening reactions.

Chapter 3

Using Antihistamines and Decongestants

In This Chapter

- Getting a grip on pharmacology
- Choosing antihistamines
- Understanding decongestants
- Surveying combination products

You can take avoidance measures and allergy-proof your home and office to significantly improve your quality of life by decreasing your exposure to the substances that trigger your allergic reactions and, in most cases, your asthma episodes. However, because allergens such as pollens, molds, and dust are everywhere, complete avoidance can be difficult, if not impossible.

Fortunately, medications are available. If used properly — based on your physician's advice — medications can prevent or relieve your allergic reactions. Effectively treating those reactions is often the single most important factor in reducing — and in some cases even eliminating — many common respiratory symptoms, thus improving your asthma and your overall quality of life.

In this chapter, I focus on antihistamines, decongestants, and combination products. Check out Chapter 4 for details on nasal corticosteroids, cromolyn sodium, anticholinergic sprays, leukotriene modifiers, and medications for allergic conjunctivitis.

Getting Familiar with Pharmacology

The many drugs available for treating nasal allergies have various uses and characteristics. Some allergy medications are designed for one specific purpose, while others have more flexible uses. In general, nasal allergy medications fall into three categories of usage:

- **Preventive:** If used properly, these types of medications can keep your nasal symptoms from developing. For people who have chronic symptoms of rhinitis, allergic or nonallergic (see Chapter 1), the most effective approach is to use antihistamines (oral or nasal) and nasal corticosteroid medications preventively.
- **Stabilizing:** These drugs can often stop a reaction that's already in progress before your immune system can release potent chemical mediators of inflammation, such as histamine and leukotrienes, that produce noticeable symptoms.
- **Relief:** Most of the commonly available over-the-counter (OTC) oral antihistamines and decongestants fall into this category. Most people use them to relieve the symptoms of rhinitis after symptoms have occurred. You're usually not taking full advantage of medications, such as antihistamines and nasal corticosteroid sprays, if you only use them after your symptoms have started.

Whether prescribed or purchased OTC, a few basic types of drugs are used to treat nasal allergies, including the following:

- Antihistamines (available in various forms OTC and by prescription)
- Antihistamine nasal sprays (available by prescription only)
- Decongestants (available OTC, by prescription in oral form, or as nonprescription nasal sprays and drops)
- Combinations of antihistamine (OTC and prescription) and decongestant products (available in oral form) are also used for multisymptomatic relief, as I discuss in the section "Two for the Nose: Combination Products"
- Nasal corticosteroid sprays (available only in prescription form)
- Mast-cell stabilizer nasal sprays containing cromolyn (available OTC)
- Anticholinergic (drying) nasal sprays (available only in prescription form)

To get the most out of your treatment, take the time to know what each medication can do to relieve your symptoms. I explain the uses and benefits of antihistamines, decongestants, and combination products in this chapter. See Chapter 4 for details on nasal corticosteroids, cromolyn, and anticholinergic sprays.

An informed patient is a healthier patient. If your doctor prescribes medication for your allergic rhinitis (or any ailment), don't hesitate to inquire about the product, why it's being prescribed, and any possible side effects.

Blocking Your Histamines with Antihistamines

As the name indicates, *antihistamines* are medications (available in tablet, capsule, liquid, and nasal spray forms or by injection) that counter the effects of *histamine* — a chemical substance released by the body as the result of injury or in response to an allergen. *First-generation* (sedating) OTC antihistamines have been in use since 1942 and are frequently the first medication option for allergic rhinitis sufferers. I discuss the important differences between OTC and most newer, *second-generation* (nonsedating or less sedating) antihistamines in the section "Newer antihistamines," later in this chapter.

Both first- and second-generation antihistamines block the effects of histamine and are most effective in controlling or alleviating symptoms of sneezing, runny nose, and itchy nose, eyes, and throat. However, these medications may not reduce nasal congestion. As a result, they're frequently combined with a decongestant to relieve symptoms of congestion. In addition, antihistamines produce various side effects, depending on the type of product (OTC or prescription), dosage levels, and course of medication.

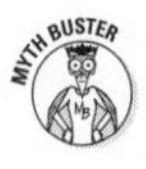

As an asthma patient, don't be afraid to use antihistamines, depending on your specific condition and your doctor's advice. In the past, product information labels advised asthma patients not to use antihistamines because these medications theoretically dry out the airways. However, studies show that the improvement of nasal symptoms produced by antihistamines improves the lung functions of many people with asthma.

Histamine hints

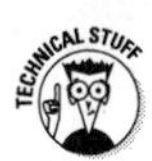

Mast cells (among the cells that line your nose and respiratory tract) produce and release a chemical substance called histamine. You may only become aware of histamine when your immune system releases massive amounts of this chemical into nasal tissue as a reaction to injury or in the presence of an allergen. After being released from the mast cells, histamine seeks out "receptor" sites located in the nasal-lining tissues.

Think of these receptors sites as locks. Histamine inserts itself like a key into the receptor site and triggers the familiar hay fever symptoms of allergic rhinitis. Antihistamines attach to the receptors before histamine gets to them. Because receptors accept only one chemical at a time, if antihistamines block histamine, allergic symptoms won't be triggered.

A dose of prevention

Many people tend to use antihistamines only as rescue medications. However, these products usually work much better and give greater relief if you take them preventively. Taking an antihistamine to relieve your symptoms is like closing the barn door after your horse has already bolted. You're not going to get that horse back (although by closing the door, you'll at least prevent any others from escaping).

Antihistamines usually work best when you take them on a regular basis before allergen exposure occurs. For example:

- If you're allergic to ragweed pollen, start using your medication at the beginning of August — before ragweed pollens are released in the middle of the month — and continue using the medication until after ragweed season is through. Even if you're exposed to significant amounts of allergen, you'll usually experience far fewer symptoms by using this type of preventive approach.

- If you know that animal dander triggers your allergic rhinitis and you plan to visit someone who has pets, take your antihistamine two to five hours beforehand. Also, remember to continue taking the antihistamine after you leave until you have an opportunity to change your clothing, because dander probably will be on your clothes.

First-generation OTC antihistamines

The most common variety of antihistamine medications is first-generation nonprescription products that are available in OTC form. Hundreds of these nonprescription antihistamine products line drugstore and supermarket shelves. Most of these products, however, are just different brand names for a few of the same active ingredients, such as:

- Brompheniramine maleate — the active ingredient in Dimetapp
- Chlorpheniramine maleate — the active ingredient in Chlor-Trimeton
- Clemastine fumarate — the active ingredient in Tavist-1
- Diphenhydramine hydrochloride — the active ingredient in Benadryl

Although first-generation OTC antihistamines can relieve allergic rhinitis symptoms, such as sneezing, runny nose, and itchy nose, eyes, and throat, they also produce side effects that can significantly interfere with your daily life. These

OTC antihistamines can cross from the bloodstream into your brain, where they affect histamine receptors in the central nervous system, resulting in drowsiness — the most serious and potentially dangerous side effect.

Consider these factors when taking nonprescription antihistamines:

- Many states in the United States consider people who take first-generation OTC antihistamines to be under the influence of drugs. The Federal Aviation Administration (FAA) prohibits pilots from flying if they take OTC antihistamines within 24 hours of flight time. Similar restrictions on the use of first-generation OTC antihistamines apply to truck and bus drivers and operators in other transportation industries.
- Operating heavy machinery or engaging in activities that require alertness, coordination, dexterity, or quick reflexes while taking first-generation OTC antihistamines is dangerous.
- Avoid alcohol, sedatives, antidepressants, or other types of tranquilizers while taking first-generation OTC antihistamines.
- First-generation OTC antihistamines can also produce other side effects, including dizziness, dryness of mouth and sinus passages, gastrointestinal irritation or distress, nasal stuffiness, and urine retention (which can aggravate existing prostate problems).
- Recent studies show that children with allergic rhinitis who take diphenhydramine (the active ingredient in Benadryl) for their symptoms score significantly lower on learning-ability tests than children who receive equivalent doses of loratadine (the second-generation OTC antihistamine Claritin).

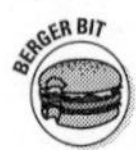

In my experience, many asthma patients don't tolerate the side effects of first-generation nonprescription antihistamines. As a result, they're less likely to take a long-term or even midterm preventive course of a first-generation nonprescription antihistamine medication. Instead, patients may resort to these older OTC antihistamines as quick, short-term fixes after allergens trigger their allergic rhinitis symptoms. This approach often leads to a pattern of debilitating, recurring symptoms that can increase the chances that asthma patients' respiratory ailments will worsen and thus diminish their quality of life.

Newer antihistamines

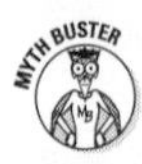

Many people assume that OTC medications are somehow safer than prescription products. In the case of antihistamines, however, the reverse may be true. Due to significant advances in research since the development of first-generation antihistamines more than 50 years ago, several of the newer, second-generation antihistamines have fewer side effects. (However, the majority of the existing prescription antihistamines are still of the older, first-generation type, and just like all the first-generation OTC antihistamines, they can potentially cause drowsiness.) Some of the benefits of these newer second-generation medications include

- Not crossing the blood-brain barrier, which means that second-generation products are nonsedating, such as fexofenadine (Allegra), loratadine (Alavert and Claritin) — reclassified by the FDA as an OTC product in 2002 — and desloratadine (Clarinex), or cause only mild sedative effects, as in the case of cetirizine (Zyrtec).

- Side effects other than drowsiness, such as dry mouth, constipation, urine retention, or blurred vision, occur less frequently or are much less noticeable with second-generation antihistamines.
- Although second-generation antihistamines, whether prescription or OTC (such as loratadine — the active ingredient in Alavert and Claritin), can cost more than most first-generation nonprescription antihistamine products, the more recently developed products work longer and require only one or two doses per day to prevent or relieve allergic rhinitis symptoms.
- For the most part, second-generation products work as rapidly as the first-generation drugs. For example, desloratadine (Clarinex), loratadine (Claritin), and cetirizine (Zyrtec) usually start functioning within 30 minutes.
- Overall, patients who use second-generation antihistamines usually experience much less disruption or impairment in their daily lives.

Because of these factors, second-generation antihistamines (see Table 3-1) can greatly improve the treatment of allergic rhinitis. In my experience, asthma patients are far more likely to stick with second-generation antihistamines for the prescribed course, which often results in a more effective prevention of allergic rhinitis symptoms and a significant improvement of their respiratory symptoms and overall condition.

Table 3-1 Second-Generation Prescription (and OTC) Antihistamines

Active Ingredient	*Formulation*	*Brand Name*	*Total Usual Daily Dose for Children under 12 Years (See Formulation Details)*	*Total Usual Daily Adult Dose*
Cetirizine	5 mg, 10 mg tablet (ages 12 years and older), syrup, 5 mg per teaspoon (2–5 years)	Zyrtec	Syrup, ½ teaspoon (2.5 mg) once per day for ages 2–5 years; 1–2 teaspoons (5–10 mg) once per day for ages 6–11 years	1 tablet once per day
Cetirizine (with 120 mg pseudo-ephedrine)	5 mg tablet (12 years and older)	Zyrtec-D	Not approved for children under 12 years of age	1 tablet twice per day
Desloratadine	5 mg tablet	Clarinex	Not approved for children under 12 years of age	1 tablet once per day

Active Ingredient	Formulation	Brand Name	Total Usual Daily Dose for Children under 12 Years (See Formulation Details)	Total Usual Daily Adult Dose
Fexofenadine	30 mg tablet (6–11 years)	Allegra-Pediatric	1 tablet twice per day	Not applicable
Fexofenadine	60 mg capsule, 60 mg tablet (12 years and older)	Allegra	Not approved for children under 12 years of age	1 capsule twice per day
Fexofenadine	180 mg tablet (12 years and older)	Allegra-24 Hour	Not approved for children under 12 years of age	1 tablet once per day
Fexofenadine (with 120 mg pseudoephedrine)	60 mg tablet (12 years and older)	Allegra-D	Not approved for children under 12 years of age	1 tablet twice per day

(continued)

Table 3-1 ***(continued)***

Active Ingredient	***Formulation***	***Brand Name***	***Total Usual Daily Dose for Children under 12 Years (See Formulation Details)***	***Total Usual Daily Adult Dose***
Loratadine	10 mg tablet (6 years and older)	Claritin	1 tablet once per day (6 years and older)	1 tablet once per day
Loratadine	10 mg tablet (rapidly disintegrating) (6 years and older)	Claritin RediTabs	1 tablet once per day (6 years and older)	1 tablet once per day
Loratadine	10 mg tablet (rapidly disintegrating) (6 years and older)	Alavert	1 tablet once per day (6 years and older)	1 tablet once per day
Loratadine (with 120 mg pseudo-ephedrine)	5 mg tablet (12 years and older)	Claritin-D 12 Hour	Not approved for children under 12 years of age	1 tablet twice per day

Active Ingredient	*Formulation*	*Brand Name*	*Total Usual Daily Dose for Children under 12 Years (See Formulation Details)*	*Total Usual Daily Adult Dose*
Loratadine (with 240 mg pseudo-ephedrine)	10 mg tablet (12 years and older)	Claritin-D 24 Hour	Not approved for children under 12 years of age	1 tablet once per day
Loratadine	Syrup, 5 mg per teaspoon (for ages 2–11 years)	Claritin Syrup	2 teaspoons (10 mg) once per day for ages 6–11 years; 1 teaspoon (5 mg) once per day for ages 2–5 years	2 teaspoons (10 mg) once per day

(continued)

Table 3-1 ***(continued)***

Active Ingredient	*Formulation*	*Brand Name*	*Total Usual Daily Dose for Children under 12 Years (See Formulation Details)*	*Total Usual Daily Adult Dose*
The following drugs are no longer available in the United States.				
Astemizole	10 mg tablet (12 years and older)	Hismanal	Not approved for children under 12 years of age	1 tablet once per day
Terfenadine	60 mg tablet (12 years and older)	Seldane	Not approved for children under 12 years of age	1 tablet twice per day
Terfenadine (with 120 mg pseudo-ephedrine)	60 mg tablet (12 years and older)	Seldane-D	Not approved for children under 12 years of age	1 tablet twice per day

mg = milligram

When used in combination with certain systemic antifungals (such as ketoconazole), antibiotics (such as erythromycin), any medical condition that may affect liver function, and even if taken with grapefruit juice, Seldane and Hismanal (no longer available in the United States but still sold in Canada and other countries) can in rare cases produce abnormal and potentially fatal heart rhythms. Make sure that you inform your doctor about any and all medications you already take — including OTC products — when you receive a prescription for another drug.

The approval of loratadine (Alavert, Claritin) in 2002 as an OTC product may at first glance seem like great news for asthma and allergy sufferers. After all, you can buy medications formulated with loratadine right off the shelf at your local drug store, and those products now cost less than when you had to have your doctor prescribe them. However, since loratadine's OTC reclassification, many physicians are concerned about some insurers' and managed-care providers' actions to no longer provide coverage of the cost of other second-generation prescription-only antihistamines.

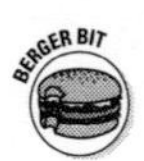

The problem with the bottom-line approach is that patients and their conditions vary widely. In some cases, even though loratadine may be the least expensive second-generation antihistamine available, it may not be the most effective drug for preventing and relieving your allergy symptoms. For this reason, both the American College of Allergy, Asthma, and Immunology (ACAAI) and the American Academy of Allergy, Asthma, and Immunology (AAAAI), which are national organizations of allergists and immunologists dedicated to quality patient care through research, advocacy, and public education, issued a statement in November 2002 concerning limited insurance coverage for second-generation antihistamines.

That statement points out that these cost-cutting attempts will reduce access to treatment for millions of patients with asthma and allergies and will also have a negative effect on the health and safety of the general public. If your doctor determines that the most effective drug for your allergies is a second-generation prescription antihistamine (such as Allegra, Clarinex, or Zyrtec), you shouldn't have to worry whether your health plan will cover the cost of that medication. In essence, the ACAAI and AAAAI are trying to make sure that you and your physician will make the decisions about your health in the exam room instead of number crunchers in HMO boardrooms.

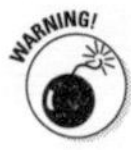

As part of their cost-cutting efforts, some managed-care organizations experiment with a dosing schedule that consists of prescribing a nonsedating second-generation antihistamine during the day and a less expensive, sedating OTC antihistamine at night. Although the concept may seem logical in theory, the reality can actually cause many problems. Because antihistamines continue to act in the body for a long time, the sedative side effects of the first-generation product may persist during the day. Studies show that using a first-generation product at night leads to sedation, performance impairment, and decreased alertness the next day.

Antihistamines and children

Treating children with any type of illness can be quite a challenge, and allergic rhinitis is certainly no exception. Besides the difficulty of getting children to actually take medications, parents also need to be concerned about side effects. In this regard, some of the second-generation antihistamines, such as the following, can be especially useful when treating children with allergic rhinitis:

- **Loratadine (Claritin):** Your doctor can prescribe this medication in a once-a-day, kid-friendly syrup or rapidly disintegrating tablet form (Alavert, Claritin RediTabs) for children as young as 6 years.
- **Cetirizine (Zyrtec):** Your doctor can prescribe this medicine for children as young as 2 years in a once-a-day syrup form.

Antihistamine nasal sprays

On the front lines of allergic rhinitis treatment, a recent addition to the antihistamine arsenal in the United States is *azelastine hydrochloride.* The FDA approved azelastine for use as a nasal spray under the product name Astelin. Remember these basic facts about this nasal spray:

- Azelastine hydrochloride is highly effective for the treatment of seasonal allergic rhinitis symptoms, such as sneezing, runny nose, and itchy nose, eyes, and throat.
- In contrast to most oral antihistamines, studies show that azelastine often helps reduce nasal congestion (stuffy nose), which may make it particularly useful in dealing with the congestion that often accompanies allergic rhinitis due to late-phase reactions.
- You can use azelastine nasal spray in combination therapy with nasal corticosteroid sprays or oral antihistamines in cases that require greater prevention or relief. (See Chapter 4 for more information on nasal corticosteroid sprays.)
- The recommended dosage for azelastine is two sprays in each nostril twice a day for patients older than 12 years and one spray in each nostril twice a day for children ages 5 to 11 years.

- The spray usually starts to take effect within three hours.
- The FDA approved azelastine hydrochloride for the treatment of *vasomotor rhinitis* (nonallergic rhinitis; see Chapter 1) for ages 12 years and older. The recommended dosage is two sprays in each nostril twice a day.
- Side effects may include a bitter taste and drowsiness in cases of prolonged use.

Decongesting Your Nose

People commonly use decongestants to relieve their stuffy noses. You can find decongestants in two forms: systemic decongestants in tablet, capsule, or liquid forms, and decongestants in the form of nasal sprays or nose drops. Unlike antihistamines, no second-generation decongestants have yet been developed.

Oral decongestants

Nonprescription oral decongestants are among the most widely used OTC products in the world, and you can find them in various tablet, capsule, and liquid forms. These medications work by shrinking blood vessels, thus reducing the amount of fluid that leaks into tissues lining the nose, thereby decreasing nasal congestion. The most commonly used decongestants are pseudoephedrine and phenylephrine.

Pseudoephedrine is the most frequently used active ingredient in OTC oral decongestants such as Sudafed and in antihistamine-decongestant combinations such as Actifed and Dimetapp. This drug is the "D" (standing for decongestant) in the commonly used second-generation products known as Allegra-D, Claritin-D, and Zyrtec-D.

Remember the following information before using this type of decongestant:

- Systemic decongestants are often combined with other drugs, such as antihistamines, *antipyretics* (fever reducers), *analgesics* (pain relievers), *antitussives* (cough suppressants), or expectorants, to provide multisymptom relief for headaches, fever, cough, sleeplessness, and other symptoms of the common cold, flu, allergic rhinitis, and other ailments.
- Oral forms of systemic decongestants can cause side effects, such as sleeplessness, nervous agitation, loss of appetite, dryness of mouth and sinuses, difficulty urinating, high blood pressure, and heart palpitations if used consistently over a long period of time.

  If you have a medical condition, such as arrhythmia, coronary heart disease, hypertension, hyperthyroidism, glaucoma, diabetes, enlarged prostate, or urinary dysfunction, don't take any product containing a decongestant (even OTC) without first checking with your doctor.
- Because of the stimulant effect of oral decongestants, use them cautiously with children. (Believe it or not, most of the parents in my practice aren't interested in unduly stimulating their kids.)

Nasal decongestants

Nonprescription decongestant nasal sprays and nose drops can provide quick and effective short-term relief of nasal congestion. However, only use them occasionally and not for more than three to five days in a row, because long-term or consistent use can result in adverse effects such as *nasal rebound* (see the nearby sidebar of the same name).

Nasal rebound

No, nasal rebound isn't a new basketball technique. This condition, more formally known as *rhinitis medicamentosa,* results from prolonged overuse of OTC decongestant nasal sprays and drops. Overusing such medications can irritate and inflame the mucous membranes in your nose more than before you used the spray, leading to more serious nasal congestion.

Unfortunately, some people increase their use of the product as their congestion worsens, leading to a vicious cycle in which more use produces more congestion. When this happens, higher doses don't clear the congestion — they only make it worse. To break this vicious cycle, stop using your OTC decongestant. Your doctor may also need to prescribe a short course of oral and/or nasal corticosteroids to clear your nasal congestion and allow you to tolerate the discontinuation of the OTC decongestant.

Remember that the warning on the label that directs you not to use the nasal decongestant spray or drops longer than three to five days really means three to five days and no more. If your stuffy nose persists beyond this point, consider using an oral decongestant.

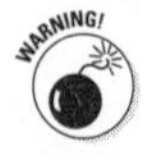

Never use decongestant nasal sprays and drops with children under the age of 6 without a doctor's supervision. If you use them properly, OTC decongestants generally produce few side effects other than occasional sneezing and dry nasal passages. The most common OTC decongestant drugs and brand-name medications include

- Naphazoline, found in Privine
- Oxymetazoline, found in Afrin, Allerest, Dristan Long Lasting, and Sinex Long Lasting

- Phenylephrine, found in Neo-Synephrine, Sinex, and Little Noses (one-eighth percent formula for infants and children)
- Xylometazoline, found in Otrivin

The dosage levels and usage frequency of these medications vary depending on each product's formulation and method of application. As always, carefully read all product instructions and warnings before using any medication.

The long-lasting products require no more than two doses a day to remain effective, but other short-acting products may work for only one to four hours. Therefore, you may need to apply short-acting products several times a day, as long as you don't exceed safe dosage levels and don't use the product continuously without checking first with your physician.

Two for the Nose: Combination Products

Antihistamines and decongestants can often be more effective in treating the full range of allergic rhinitis symptoms if you combine them in one preparation. You can find numerous oral OTC combination products in tablet, capsule, and liquid forms on store shelves.

An antihistamine, such as chlorpheniramine or brompheniramine, is often combined with a decongestant, such as pseudoephedrine. These products are also frequently combined with other active ingredients — pain relievers, cough suppressants, and fever relievers, for example — to provide relief for a variety of ailments, such as cold and flu symptoms.

The onset of action and dosage frequency vary with different products. Tablets and capsules generally come in two varieties:

- **Rapid release:** These medications start working quickly but usually lose effectiveness within four hours.
- **Sustained release:** As you may expect, these products work the opposite way; they act slower but last longer than rapid release medications — usually six to eight hours or longer.

Nondrowsy OTC formulas may contain pain relievers, fever reducers, cough suppressants, or other active ingredients for multisymptom relief but don't contain first-generation antihistamines, which cause drowsiness. Therefore, these formulas don't usually provide relief from the sneezing, runny nose, and itchy nose, eyes, and throat that are significant symptoms of allergic rhinitis.

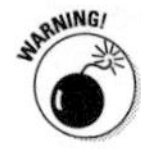

The decongestant in combination products can still cause sleeplessness, nervous agitation, loss of appetite, dryness of mouth and sinuses, high blood pressure, and heart palpitations, especially in older patients. Likewise, the antihistamine in combination products can still cause drowsiness. For example, the antihistamine diphenhydramine (Benadryl) is the active ingredient in many popular sleep aids, such as Nytol. See the following section for more details.

Analyzing the upside and downside

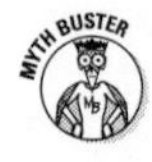

Because of their sedative effects, OTC antihistamines are generally thought of as *downers.* Likewise, because decongestants act as stimulants, they're considered *uppers.* You may think that combining these two types of drugs in a single OTC product cancels out both the sedative and stimulant side effects. However, a person may experience both the upper and downer effects at the same time — the worst of both worlds, in other words — resulting in an agitated, jittery form of drowsiness.

If my patient's condition warrants a combination product, I usually prescribe a nonsedating antihistamine formulated with a decongestant, such as Allegra-D, or possibly a less sedating antihistamine formulated with a decongestant, such as Zyrtec-D. The decongestant (pseudoephedrine) in these products usually doesn't produce as great a stimulant effect as other decongestants, such as phenylpropanolamine, which the FDA recently removed from the market. As a result, the patient gets the benefits of both a nonsedating antihistamine and a less stimulating decongestant action, minimizing the adverse downer or upper side effects.

Most OTC liquid forms are short-acting, which means that they usually require up to four doses a day. However, you may prefer to use liquids, especially syrup forms that often contain flavorings (and sometimes sweeteners), to treat children as well as adults who have trouble swallowing tablets and capsules. Another option in these cases is to use prescription chewable formulations of these products, such as AH-Chew Chewable Tablets.

One size fits all may not suit your condition

Although combination antihistamine and decongestant products may work well when you need quick relief, the products are less viable for long-term use because you can't adjust the dosage levels of the individual active ingredients. Each dose, whether in tablet, capsule, or liquid form, delivers the same amount of antihistamine and decongestant (as well as other active ingredients) to your system whether you need relief from one symptom or the full range of ailments.

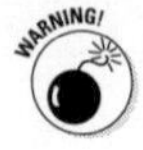

If you're considering switching combination products because the one you use doesn't seem effective, check the active ingredients on other medications to make sure that you don't buy the same antihistamine and decongestant combination under a different brand name.

Chapter 4

Relieving Allergies with Other Medications

In This Chapter

- Understanding nasal corticosteroids
- Looking at cromolyn sodium
- Using anticholinergic sprays
- Getting the scoop on leukotriene modifiers
- Easing itchy, red eyes

Medications can prevent or relieve your allergic reactions when they're used properly (based on your physician's advice). In this chapter, I explain the use of nasal corticosteroids, cromolyn sodium, anticholinergic sprays, leukotriene modifiers, and medications for allergic conjunctivitis. See Chapter 3 for details about other medications that relieve allergies, such as antihistamines, decongestants, and combination products.

Using Nasal Corticosteroids

The most effective medication currently available for controlling the four major symptoms of allergic rhinitis — sneezing, itching, runny nose, and nasal congestion — is *nasal corticosteroid spray.* Patients and the general public commonly refer to these corticosteroid products as *steroids,* or *cortisone.* However, in this book, I use the proper term *corticosteroid* for these types of nasal sprays to avoid confusion.

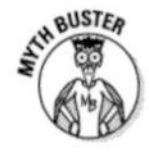

The negative perception that some people have of steroids is mostly due to attempts by some athletes to build up muscle mass by abusing *anabolic steroids.* In fact, the types of steroids used in corticosteroid nasal sprays are a completely different type of drug than anabolic steroids (which are actually male hormones).

The spray is available by prescription only and is administered by an *aqueous* (non-CFC propellant) mechanical pump. The following information can help you and your doctor decide whether nasal corticosteroids can work for you:

- Nasal corticosteroid sprays suppress the inflammation of nasal passages, thereby clearing your nose for easier breathing.
- Nasal corticosteroid sprays are most effective if you use them daily as preventive medications. For a guide to safe dosage levels, see Table 4-1.

  Never exceed dosage levels with these products to minimize the possibility of the medication causing systemic side effects, such as those associated with oral corticosteroids.

Table 4-1 Nasal Corticosteroid Sprays

Active Ingredient	*Formulation*	*Brand Name*	*Total Usual Daily Dose for Children under 12 Years (See Formulation Details)*	*Total Usual Daily Adult Dose*
Beclomethasone	42 mcg per inhalation	Beconase AQ, Vancenase AQ	1–2 sprays each nostril twice per day (6–11 years)	1–2 sprays each nostril twice per day
Beclomethasone	84 mcg per inhalation	Vancenase AQ Double Strength	1–2 sprays each nostril once per day (6–11 years)	1–2 sprays each nostril once per day
Budesonide	32 mcg per inhalation	Rhinocort Aqua	1–4 sprays each per day (6–11 years)	1–2 sprays each nostril once per day

(continued)

Table 4-1 *(continued)*

Active Ingredient	*Formulation*	*Brand Name*	*Total Usual Daily Dose for Children under 12 Years (See Formulation Details)*	*Total Usual Daily Adult Dose*
Flunisolide	25 mcg per inhalation	Nasarel, Nasalide	1 spray each nostril three times per day or 2 sprays each nostril twice per day (6–11 years)	2 sprays each nostril twice per day
Fluticasone	50 mcg per inhalation	Flonase	1 spray each nostril once per day; may be increased to 2 sprays each nostril once per day (4–11 years)	2 sprays each nostril once per day or 1 spray each nostril twice per day; may be decreased to maintenance dose of 1 spray each nostril once per day

Active Ingredient	*Formulation*	*Brand Name*	*Total Usual Daily Dose for Children under 12 Years (See Formulation Details)*	*Total Usual Daily Adult Dose*
Mometasone	50 mcg per inhalation	Nasonex	1 spray each nostril once per day; may be increased to 2 sprays each nostril once per day (3– 11 years)	2 sprays each nostril once per day
Triamcinolone	55 mcg per inhalation	Nasacort AQ	2 sprays each nostril nostril once per day (6–11 years)	2 sprays each once per day

mcg = microgram

- Nasal corticosteroid sprays provide gradual relief of allergic rhinitis symptoms. Initially, you may need to use the medication for several days before the spray suppresses the inflammation. Full effectiveness may require two to three weeks of daily application.
- Only use nasal corticosteroids if your nose is clear enough for the spray to penetrate. If your nose is seriously congested, you may need to use a nasal decongestant for only the first three to five days just prior to administering the nasal corticosteroid spray. See Chapter 3 for details on nasal decongestants.
- In order to prevent injuring your *septum* (the bone that divides the nose into two nostrils), direct the spray away from the septum and slightly in the direction of your ears. You may even want to spray the product once in the air to judge the force of the spray before using it in your nose.
- Using an aqueous (AQ) formulation of a nasal corticosteroid, because of its gentler action on the nasal lining, can often minimize the typical adverse side effects of nasal corticosteroid sprays, such as nasal irritation, burning, drying, and nosebleeds.

Although some evidence indicates that nasal corticosteroid sprays are highly effective and safe for children, some doctors are concerned about the possible effects the sprays may temporarily have on the growth rate of children who use them. If your child uses a nasal corticosteroid spray, make sure that your child's physician knows about your concerns so he can accurately monitor your youngster's growth.

Steroids to avoid

Although nasal corticosteroid sprays are highly effective and generally safe for both adults and children when administered under a physician's care, using other forms of steroids is less advisable and potentially unsafe. The following steroids are potentially harmful to you:

- **Oral corticosteroids:** I advise using quick bursts of short-acting oral steroids (such as prednisone or methylprednisolone) only in cases of severe nasal rebound or nasal polyps, where a decongestant nasal spray can't penetrate sufficiently to decongest your nose. In such cases, you may require a short course of oral corticosteroids to sufficiently clear your congestion so that you can use a nasal corticosteroid spray.
- **Intranasal injections:** Cortisone shots into the nose aren't appropriate treatment for allergic rhinitis because of their potential for serious side effects, including vision disturbances and possibly even blindness.

Cromolyn Sodium

Cromolyn sodium, an anti-inflammatory OTC nasal spray, may be highly effective in controlling symptoms of allergic rhinitis when you use it properly. (You can find this medicine under the brand name Nasalcrom.) Cromolyn sodium stabilizes mast cells, thereby preventing the release of histamine and other chemical mediators that can cause nasal inflammation.

To help determine whether cromolyn sodium nasal spray might work for you, check out these facts about its recommended use and effectiveness:

- Cromolyn sodium is most effective if you start using it two to four weeks before exposure to allergens. In cases of occupational allergic rhinitis or of limited exposure to allergens, using the spray immediately prior to an isolated, single, allergen exposure (before mowing the lawn or visiting a home with pet), if your nasal passages aren't already congested, may also provide some relief.
- If allergic rhinitis symptoms are already present, you may need a short course of a combination antihistamine-decongestant for the first few days that you use cromolyn sodium. (See Chapter 3 for details on combination products.)
- Because cromolyn sodium has an excellent safety profile and produces no significant side effects, doctors may often prescribe it for children and pregnant women.
- You can purchase cromolyn sodium in a metered spray form. The recommended dosage for adults and children older than 6 years is one spray in each nostril, three to six times per day at regular intervals. Only administer cromolyn sodium to children between 2 and 6 years of age under the supervision of a doctor.

Reducing Mucus with Anticholinergic Sprays

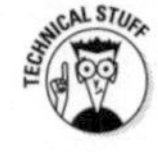

Ipratropium bromide is the active ingredient in the anticholinergic products (drying agents) that sell under the brand name Atrovent Nasal Spray. As the name of this drug class indicates, anticholinergics counter cholinergic activity by blocking *acetylcholine* — a neurotransmitter that stimulates mucus production — from attaching to chemical receptors in the nose. Therefore, these sprays reduce the amount of mucus in your nose.

Some basic facts about anticholinergic sprays include the following:

- Ipratropium bromide effectively reduces runny nose, as seen in conditions such as *vasomotor* (nonallergic) rhinitis (see the nearby "Skier's nose" sidebar) or the common cold.
- Ipratropium bromide has little effect on other allergic rhinitis symptoms, such as stuffy nose, sneezing, or itchy nose.
- Your doctor can prescribe Atrovent Nasal Spray in two strengths — 0.03 percent for relief of runny nose associated with allergic and nonallergic rhinitis in adults and children older than 6 years and 0.06 percent for relief of runny nose associated with the common cold in adults and children older than 12 years.
- Spray two sprays per nostril two to three times per day (0.03 percent) or three or four times per day (0.06 percent) at regular intervals for the recommended dosage.

Skier's nose

Ever notice how often skiers blow their noses? When I was training at National Jewish Hospital in Denver, I managed to get to the ski slopes occasionally. When I did, I noticed many boxes of tissues at the bottom of the ski lifts. As I discovered, the tissue boxes were there because of what people call *skier's nose,* which is triggered by cold air and is symptomatic of vasomotor rhinitis (see Chapter 1).

(continued)

(continued)

I've since found that Atrovent Nasal Spray works well to prevent skier's nose as well as jogger's nose if you use it before being exposed to cold air, and it also works well for treatment after symptoms appear. However, doctors also use anticholinergic eye drops similar to ipratropium bromide (the active ingredient) to dilate patients' eyes, so make sure that you keep the spray away from your eyes, or you won't see that mogul coming right at you.

Treating Rhinitis with Leukotriene Modifiers

Leukotrienes play a significant role in asthma attacks. These chemicals, found in the mast cells that line the airways of the lungs and nose, enhance mucus production, constrict the bronchial passages, and promote further inflammation of the respiratory lining by attracting additional inflammatory cells into the airways.

Leukotriene modifiers, such as montelukast (Singulair) and zafirlukast (Accolate), approved for the treatment of asthma, are relatively newer drugs that competitively block leukotriene activity at the receptor site, thus decreasing the amount of mucus generated by exposure to allergens.

Studies have shown that leukotriene modifiers may effectively treat patients whose allergic rhinitis symptoms don't respond solely to antihistamines. If you're in that category, ask your doctor whether leukotriene modifiers may work for you. One of these drugs, Singulair, which the FDA recently approved for treatment of allergic rhinitis, also shows promise in treating symptoms of allergic conjunctivitis.

Keeping an Eye out for Allergic Conjunctivitis

Allergic conjunctivitis often coexists with allergic rhinitis. In fact, most of the same allergens involved in allergic rhinitis can trigger allergic conjunctivitis. Characteristic symptoms of this ailment include redness of the eyes and the underside of the eyelids and swollen, itchy, and watery eyes.

Because the mechanisms of allergic rhinitis and allergic conjunctivitis are similar, conjunctivitis is often treated with some of the same types of drugs used to control rhinitis in solutions specifically formulated for safe use in the eye. Treatment can include

- **Prescription antihistamines:** Two newer second-generation prescription antihistamines, *levocabastine* (Livostin) and *emedastine* (Emadine), appear to be more effective than OTC antihistamines for the treatment of allergic conjunctivitis. Normal recommended dosage for both of these products is one drop per eye up to four times a day for up to two weeks.
- **OTC decongestants:** Products include Clear Eyes, Clear Eyes ACR, Visine A.C., Visine L.R., Visine Moisturizing, and Visine Original.
- **Combinations of OTC antihistamines and decongestants:** Product names include Naphcon-A, Vasocon-A, Ocuhist, Prefrin, and VasoClear.
- **Mast-cell stabilizers:** This group of medications inhibits mast cells from releasing chemical mediators of inflammation, thus potentially preventing allergic symptoms from developing. These types of eye drop products include cromolyn sodium (Crolom, Opticrom), nedocromil sodium (Alocril), and lodoxamide (Alomide).

Administer cromolyn sodium on a regular basis, four times a day. For infrequent allergen exposure (when visiting someone with pets, for example), use cromolyn sodium immediately before you visit. Nedocromil sodium provides effective relief of both the early- and late-phase allergic response. The normal dosage for Alocril is one to two drops in each eye twice per day. Lodoxamide isn't approved for use specifically for allergic conjunctivitis but has shown some effectiveness in clinical trials as a treatment for vernal conjunctivitis (a chronic eye condition that can cause severe burning and intense itching and marked sensitivity to bright light).

- **Nonsteroidal anti-inflammatory drugs (NSAIDs):** Ketorolac (Acular) is a type of NSAID that can relieve the itching of seasonal allergic conjunctivitis. Normal dosage is one drop per eye, four times per day.
- **Combination antihistamine and mast-cell stabilizer:** The most recent additions to allergic conjunctivitis eye products are olapatadine (Patanol), ketotifen (Zaditor), azelastine (Optivar), and epinastine (Elestat), which are available by prescription in the United States. The normal recommended dosage for Patanol is one drop in each affected eye twice per day, at an interval of six to eight hours. For Zaditor, the recommended dosage is one drop in each eye twice daily, every eight to twelve hours. The recommended dosage for Optivar and also for Elestat is one drop in each eye twice a day.

Doctors prescribe corticosteroid eye drops for severe cases of allergic conjunctivitis that are unresponsive to the medications I describe in the preceding section. However, monitor the use of corticosteroid eye drops closely because using these products improperly can lead to very serious adverse side effects. Don't ever use corticosteroid eye drops in cases where you suspect you have a viral infection of the eyes, such as herpes, because using these products may result in prolonging the course of and increasing the severity of the viral infection. In addition, prolonged use of these corticosteroid eye drops may result in glaucoma, vision disturbances, and cataract formations. Consider consulting a qualified ophthalmologist before routinely using corticosteroid eye products.

Patients with allergic conjunctivitis should use eye drops during peak pollination seasons, in addition to their other prescribed medication for allergic rhinitis, to minimize eye discomfort. Try not to rub your eyes. Even though they may itch, rubbing them usually only makes matters worse. Instead, gently rinsing your eyes with clean water or a soothing OTC sterile irrigating solution can often wash away pollen and help relieve your symptoms.

If you experience severe allergic conjunctivitis, your doctor may prescribe an oral antihistamine, eye drops, and/or a combination of two different eye drop products for maximum relief of your symptoms.

Chapter 5

Treating Ear, Nose, and Throat Complications

In This Chapter

- Diagnosing sinus and ear infections
- Clearing the nosy road to your ears and sinuses

Because many people refer to allergic rhinitis as *hay fever,* they often think that this allergic condition is just a nuisance rather than a serious disease. However, allergic rhinitis isn't a simple problem. Allergic rhinitis is an ailment that often requires serious attention and management, not only because the symptoms can worsen your asthma and severely affect your quality of life, but also because ineffective treatment can lead to serious complications, such as *sinusitis* (an inflammation of the sinuses) and *otitis media* (an inflammation of the middle ear).

Other conditions, such as *tonsillitis* (an inflammation of the tonsils), adenoid disease, and chronic cough can also be worsened by *postnasal drip* (nasal discharge that trickles down the back of your throat). This characteristic symptom of allergic rhinitis, which usually increases in severity when the ailment is poorly managed, can result in the spread of bacteria-laden mucus that irritates and/or infects the throat's lining.

In addition, ineffectively treated allergic rhinitis and resulting postnasal drip can also adversely affect asthma patients with gastroesophageal reflux disease (GERD). This digestive disorder, which is the third most common cause of chronic cough in North America, is a trigger of asthma symptoms in a large number of asthmatics, especially in cases of nonallergic, adult-onset asthma.

This chapter explains the causes and symptoms of sinusitis and otitis media and the appropriate methods of preventing and treating these ailments.

Complicating Your Allergies: Sinusitis

If you've ever had cold or nasal symptoms that didn't seem to go away, you may have actually been suffering from a form of sinusitis. This often painful condition develops as a result of swollen nasal and sinus passages that frequently result from allergic rhinitis. Many asthma patients often confuse sinusitis symptoms with the symptoms of a cold, flu, or allergy.

Sinusitis is one of the most common health problems in the United States. Current estimates are that sinusitis affects 35 million people each year. Because of the congestion and discomfort that sinusitis causes, it's one of the most common reasons for doctor visits in the United States.

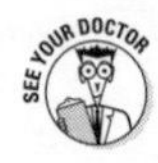

Consult a doctor as soon as you suspect you may have sinusitis. Complications, such as aggravation of asthma, recurrent bronchitis, otitis media, and nasal polyps, can occur if you manage your sinusitis poorly. Chronic sinus infections can result in swollen adenoids that may require surgery to remove. On a more positive note, studies show that asthma patients who effectively manage their sinusitis can significantly improve their respiratory symptoms.

Recognizing common causes

In a significant number of sinusitis cases, allergic rhinitis precedes the start of a sinus infection. Research shows that more than half of all children in the United States who receive treatment for sinusitis also have allergic rhinitis.

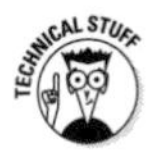

Vasomotor rhinitis, a nonallergic form of rhinitis that results from sudden temperature changes or exposure to tobacco smoke, pollutants, and other irritants (see Chapter 1), can also contribute to sinusitis. Swimmers, divers, fliers (passengers as well as flight crews), and other people with this form of rhinitis who frequently experience pressure and weather changes may be particularly prone to developing sinusitis if they don't effectively manage their rhinitis symptoms.

Factors (you may have one or more of these) that can also increase your chances of developing sinusitis are

- **Upper respiratory viral infections:** Viruses, such as those associated with the common cold, are the most frequent causes of sinusitis.
- **Bacteria:** The same family of germs that can cause acute otitis media *(Streptococcus pneumonia, Haemophilus influenza, Moraxella catarrhalis)* can cause acute bacterial sinusitis. Unlike viral infections, this type of sinusitis responds to antibiotic therapy.
- **Fungal:** This type of sinusitis infection can develop in otherwise healthy patients who have

been on long-term antibiotic treatment or have been taking oral corticosteroids on a chronic basis. *Aspergillus* is the most common fungus that causes these types of cases and is also frequently implicated in cases of *allergic fungal sinusitis.* Signs of this recurring fungal infection, which can often affect individuals with allergic rhinitis and/or asthma, are sinus infections and *nasal polyps* (growths in the nose).

- **Nasal rebound:** Overuse of OTC nasal decongestants can also predispose you to sinusitis. (See Chapter 3 for more information.)
- **Anatomical obstructions:** Nasal polyps, other growths, enlarged adenoids (particularly in children), and a deviated nasal septum (the great divide between the nostrils — see Chapter 1 for more details) can increase your chances of developing sinusitis.
- **Other diseases:** Patients with cystic fibrosis, in which abnormally thick mucus is produced and the function of the *cilia* (tiny hairlike projections of certain types of cells that sweep debris-laden mucus through the airways) is impaired, frequently suffer from sinus infections. In addition, AIDS and other immune-deficiency diseases often weaken the body's defenses to the point where bacteria and viruses can cause many types of infections, including sinusitis. These patients with compromised immune systems may be particularly vulnerable to various forms of fungal sinus infections.

Sinus science

Allergists refer to the sinuses that surround your nose — called *paranasal sinuses* — when they discuss sinusitis. *Para* is Greek for around or near; *nasal* refers to the nose; and *sinus* is Latin for a hollow place. Your sinuses are hollow cavities in the bones that surround your nasal cavity (see Figure 5-1); hence the word *sinusitis,* inflammation *(itis)* of the sinuses.

The three types of paranasal sinuses come in pairs (one on each side of the nose) and are named for the bones that house them. They include

- **Maxillary sinuses:** The largest of the sinuses, these sinuses are located in your cheekbones.
- **Frontal sinuses:** These sinuses reside in your forehead above your eyes.
- **Ethmoid sinuses:** These sinuses are immediately behind your eyes and nose.

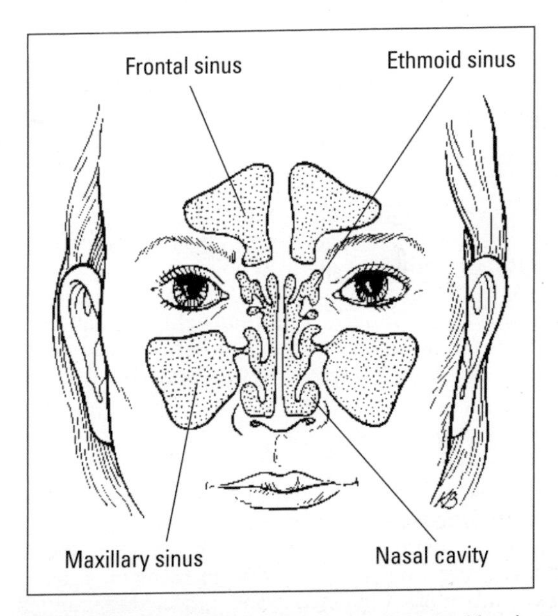

Figure 5-1: Your sinuses are actually hollow cavities that surround your nasal cavity.

The other sinus affected by sinusitis is the *sphenoid* sinus, located behind your nose near the base of your brain.

Sinus infections most often affect the maxillary, frontal, and ethmoid sinuses. The most common complication affects the orbit around the eye, causing *cellulitis* and possibly forming an *abscess* (a localized collection of pus surrounded by inflamed tissue). Patients with this type of infection may look as though they've been severely punched in the eye. Because the sphenoid sinus is near the brain, an infection in this area, although rare, is usually associated with infections in all the other sinuses *(pansinusitis)* and can have very serious consequences if infected fluids spread to the central nervous system. Untreated sinusitis has the potential to lead to life-threatening conditions, such as *meningitis* (an infection of the membranes that envelop the brain and spinal cord) and brain abscesses.

Your maxillary sinuses are present at birth, along with immature ethmoid sinuses, which begin to fully develop when you're between 3 and 7 years old. Contrary to previous medical opinion, children under 5 years can experience sinus infections that require appropriate therapy. If your young child has allergic rhinitis, effectively treating his or her condition is vital in reducing the risk of developing sinusitis.

Practical sinus

Sinuses are a vital part of your body's defense against the airborne bacteria, viruses, irritants, and allergens that you constantly inhale. Under normal circumstances, the mucus in your sinuses traps most of these intruders. Cilia sweep the particle-laden mucus through connecting *ostia* (sinus drainage openings) into your nasal passages, which then drains into your throat. From your throat, the mucus moves into your stomach, where your digestive system can neutralize and eventually eliminate the offending substances.

In addition to helping clear your upper respiratory tract of particle-laden mucus, your sinuses serve other important roles. For example, your sinuses act as:

- Air pockets that lighten your skull — otherwise, your head would be too heavy for your neck. Calling someone an airhead is actually an anatomically correct statement.
- Resonance chambers that provide space for your voice to resonate.
- Climate adjusters, warming and humidifying the air that you inhale.
- Insulators, which also warm the base of your brain, located directly behind your nose.
- Shock absorbers, protecting the inside of your skull from injury.

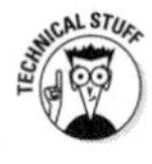

Allergic rhinitis irritates the nasal and sinus lining, causing the linings to swell, which narrows the sinus drainage openings into the nasal cavity. At the same time, your immune system's allergic response to allergic rhinitis increases mucus production. This combination of increased mucus flow and a swollen sinus lining overwhelms the cilia's abilities to sweep out the mucus, which then becomes infected.

Think of a swiftly flowing stream. If the stream dams up, the water usually stagnates and turns into a breeding ground for all sorts of organisms. The same process applies to your sinuses, which is why it's crucial to avoid letting them turn into swamps.

How long has this been goin' on?

Although no universal definition exists for the various presentations of sinusitis, most doctors base their sinusitis classifications on the duration and types of symptoms involved. Therefore, doctors often use the following terms to classify cases of sinusitis:

- **Acute sinusitis:** Symptoms of acute sinusitis persist for up to three to four weeks, although some doctors may diagnose symptoms that continue for up to eight weeks as acute.

  Typical symptoms of acute sinusitis include upper respiratory infection; runny nose with infected mucus that often appears as cloudy, thick, yellowish, or greenish nasal discharge; cloudy, yellowish, or greenish postnasal drip; facial pain or pressure around cheeks, eyes, and lower nose (mainly in adults, less commonly in children), especially while bending over or moving vigorously (for example, during exercise); nasal congestion, headache, fever, and cough; a reduction or loss of the sense of smell, pain in upper teeth or the upper jawbone, and bad breath; and in some children, nausea and vomiting due to gagging on infected mucus.
- **Chronic sinusitis:** When your condition lasts longer than four weeks, doctors usually consider you a chronic sufferer. In many cases, chronic sinusitis can last for months with combinations of the same symptoms as acute sinusitis, although you may not have a fever. For this reason, many people with chronic sinusitis think that they suffer from frequent or constant colds.
- **Recurrent sinusitis:** Doctors usually define recurrent sinusitis as three or more episodes of acute sinusitis per year. The recurring episodes may occur as a result of different causes. If you have recurrent sinusitis, your doctor may refer you to

an allergist to determine whether allergies are the underlying cause of your condition. (See Chapter 2 for more details on allergy testing.)

Diagnosing sinusitis

Often, your doctor can diagnose sinusitis based on your symptoms and medical history. Your doctor may ask questions like the following:

- When did you first notice your symptoms?
- What hurts? Where do you feel the pain?
- Does your family have a history of allergies and sinus problems?
- What have you done to treat your symptoms? What sorts of medications have you taken, and what has been their effect?

Your doctor also conducts a physical exam of your nose and sinuses in order to confirm diagnosis. This exam may include

- Taking your temperature to check for fever and listening to your chest to see whether the infection has spread to your lungs.
- Lightly tapping your forehead and cheekbones to check for sensitivity in your frontal and maxillary sinuses.
- Looking for infected mucus in your nose and the back of your throat. This exam may require insertion of a flexible fiber-optic device, known as an *endoscope* or a fiber-optic rhinoscope, so that your doctor can clearly view potentially infected areas.

Your doctor may use sophisticated imaging techniques to confirm the diagnosis of sinusitis. *Computed tomography* (CT) is currently the gold standard and, in many cases, is replacing the use of less-accurate sinus X-rays. A CT scan, also known as a *CAT scan,* is a diagnostic test that combines the use of X-rays with state-of-the-art computer technology. This test uses a series of X-ray beams from many different angles to create cross-sectional images of your body — in this case, of your head and sinuses. With computer assistance, these images are assembled into a three-dimensional picture that can display organs, bones, and tissues in great detail.

Determining the best course of treatment

To effectively treat your sinusitis, you need to effectively manage your allergic rhinitis. In many cases, appropriately treating your allergic rhinitis also improves your sinusitis. Avoidance and allergy-proofing are crucial tools you can use to effectively treat your allergies. Chapters 3 and 4 provide you with an in-depth explanation of allergy medications that you may find appropriate for your condition.

In addition to addressing your allergic rhinitis, doctors can also prescribe a variety of treatments for sinusitis, ranging from medication to irrigation to surgery.

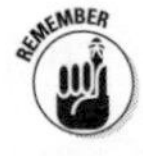

Antibiotics are the most common medications that doctors prescribe to clear up the bacterial (not viral) infection in your sinuses. When taking antibiotics, keep the following in mind:

- Because the blood flow to your sinuses is poor, you may need to take your prescribed antibiotics for a while before you notice a beneficial effect. However, most cases of acute sinusitis respond to antibiotic treatment within two weeks.

- In cases of chronic sinusitis, don't be surprised if your doctor prescribes a six- to eight-week course of antibiotic therapy with combined use of intranasal steroids (see Chapter 4) to eliminate your bacterial infection.
- In some cases of acute or chronic sinusitis, you may notice a sudden improvement in your symptoms soon after you start a course of antibiotics, and you may consider stopping the medication at that point. However, take the complete course of antibiotics to ensure that all the bacteria have been completely eliminated.

In addition to prescribing antibiotics to clear up the bacterial infection in your sinuses, your doctor may also prescribe medications to treat symptoms of allergic rhinitis (see Chapters 3 and 4).

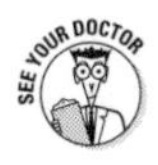

Your doctor may advise you to use a nasal douche cup, nasal spray bottle, nasal bulb syringe, Water Pik with nasal attachment, or some other type of nasal wash device to irrigate your nostrils with warm saline solution. You can use these devices at home to relieve pressure and congestion in your nasal passages. Ask your doctor for specific instructions on how to use nasal wash devices.

Your doctor may also advise a simple home remedy to help clear your sinuses and relieve discomfort, which consists of inhaling steam to liquefy and soften crusty mucus while moisturizing your inflamed passages.

Use the following method for inhaling steam:

1. **Boil water in a kettle on the stove.**
2. **Carefully pour the boiling water in a pan or basin on a low table.**

3. **Sit at the table and drape a towel over your head, leaning over the pan or basin to form a kind of human tent with your head as the pole.**
4. **Hold your face a few inches above the steaming water and breathe the steam through your nose for approximately ten minutes.**

Two steam treatments a day may provide relief. However, you still need to deal with the underlying cause of the sinus infection, so I don't advise relying solely on this home remedy as the only therapy for your infectious sinusitis.

If other treatment methods don't provide effective relief, you may need surgery, especially if physical obstructions, such as a deviated septum or nasal polyps, contribute to your condition. However, if allergic rhinitis is the underlying cause of your sinusitis, surgery alone won't resolve your sinus problems. You must continue managing your allergic rhinitis to avoid further complications. By the same token, treating your allergies alone won't reverse the damage that sinusitis may have already caused.

If your doctor thinks that surgery is advisable, she'll refer you to an ear, nose, and throat specialist, or ENT, known as an *otolaryngologist* (remember that word for your next Scrabble game — you could score big). Before you consider surgery, make sure your doctor thoroughly reviews your medical history and evaluates your clinical condition.

Never hesitate to ask your surgeon for further information concerning your planned surgical procedure, such as how long the procedure takes, where and when it will be performed, any possible complications that may occur, and how soon you can get back to work or school.

The good news about surgery for your sinuses is that the two most common procedures are minimally invasive. An ENT specialist can perform them on an outpatient basis with local anesthesia, although he may use general anesthesia in certain cases. The two procedures most often used are

- **Antral puncture and irrigation:** This procedure opens up your sinuses so they can drain and irrigate properly but is used less often now since the advent of fiber-optic surgery.
- **Functional endoscopic sinus surgery:** This procedure is more complex than antral puncture and irrigation. Functional endoscopic sinus surgery often involves enlarging the ethmoid and maxillary sinus openings into the nasal cavity and removing and cleaning the infected sinus membranes, resulting in improved drainage. This procedure reestablishes the ventilation of your ethmoid, maxillary, and frontal sinuses. Otolaryngologists perform this type of surgery with high-tech computer-assisted instruments and navigation devices to ensure pinpoint accuracy.

An ounce of prevention . . .

If you have allergic rhinitis, consider taking the following preventive measures to keep your sinuses clear if you come down with an upper respiratory infection (such as the common cold) or experience an allergy attack:

- **Take the appropriate medications.** See Chapters 3 and 4 for a complete listing.
- **Drink plenty of water.** Water keeps your mucus thin and fluid so your sinuses can drain more easily.

- **Be nice to your nose.** Blow it gently, preferably one nostril at a time.
- **Avoid flying.** If you have to travel by air while you have a cold or an allergy attack, use a topical nasal decongestant spray prior to takeoff. The spray prevents the sudden pressure changes from blocking your sinuses and ears.
- **Avoid swimming.** You probably won't feel like going to the beach or the pool if you have a cold or allergy attack, and your sinuses won't enjoy the pressure changes that swimming and diving involve (scuba diving isn't a good idea either).

Otitis Media

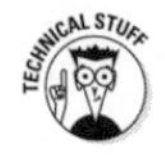

Otitis media is an inflammation of the middle ear as well as a condition in which fluid accumulates in your ear. This condition is in contrast to *otitis externa,* which affects the external auditory canal, known commonly as *swimmer's ear.* Based on the definitions I provide of sinusitis and rhinitis (see Chapter 1), you can probably already guess what *otitis* means: an inflammation *(itis)* of the ear (*otikos* in Greek). *Media* means middle, by the way. Infectious organisms, such as bacteria and viruses, often affect the middle ear. Otitis media can often develop as a result of allergic rhinitis and from complications of sinusitis.

Middle ear infections and fluid in the ear are especially common in young children and infants. In fact, otitis media is the most common reason in the United States for pediatric visits, with doctors treating at least 10 million children annually for ear infections. Otitis media can have serious consequences for youngsters, in particular by adversely affecting a child's development and learning ability due to potential hearing loss.

The most common forms of otitis media are

- **Acute otitis media (AOM):** This condition involves inflammation and infection of the middle ear and Eustachian tube. The peak incidence is between 6 months and 1 year of age, decreasing with age and with fewer episodes after 7 years of age.
- **Otitis media with effusion (OME):** Doctors also refer to this condition as *serous otitis media* — fluid in the middle ear. This condition, which occurs commonly in children ages 2 to 7 years, can lead to hearing loss if not treated properly.

Revealing common causes

In a significant number of cases, allergic rhinitis precedes an ear infection. A long-term study of 2,000 children found that 50 percent of the patients with chronic and recurrent ear infections who were 3 years of age and older had allergic rhinitis. Other conditions that can increase your chances of developing ear infections include

- Sinusitis. The same factors that can lead to sinus infections, such as exposure to allergens, tobacco smoke, pollutants, and other irritants, can also contribute to ear infections.
- Enlarged adenoids.
- Unrepaired cleft palate.
- Nasal polyps.
- Pacifier use by babies.
- Defective or immature immune system.
- Benign or malignant tumors.

- Teething. Some physicians believe that teething in young children can also contribute to ear infections, but no one has established a direct connection.

Many of the conditions in the previous list affect infants and young children. Always ask your physician to check your child's ear for infection and fluid in the middle ear anytime he or she is ill.

Getting an earful

The visible part of your ear — that funny-looking protrusion on the side of your head — is only the tip of the iceberg. Most of your ears' functions take place inside your skull in chambers, tubes, and passages that register and conduct sound and also provide your sense of balance. Figure 5-2 shows the parts that make up the ear.

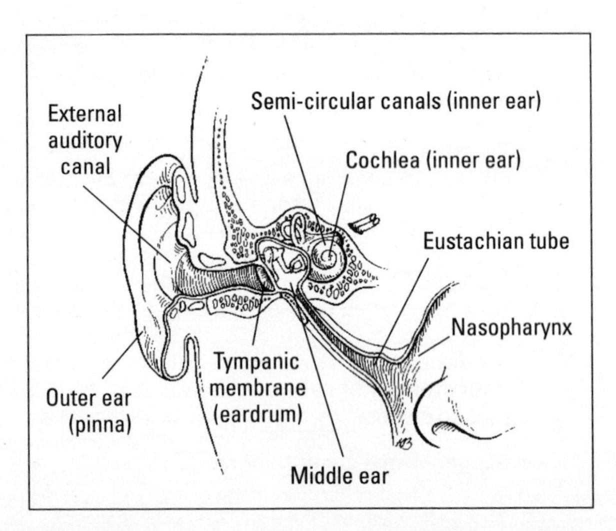

Figure 5-2: See how the less visible part of your ear appears.

- **Outer ear:** Also known as the *pinna,* this structure is what many people think of as the ear. The primary function of this skin-covered flap of cartilage is to funnel sound into the middle ear.
- **Middle ear:** This air-filled chamber is bordered by the *tympanic membrane* (commonly known as the *eardrum*) and small bones that enable your eardrum to function. Through its connection (the *Eustachian tube*) to the *nasopharynx* (back of the nose), your middle ear also equalizes the air pressure on both sides of your eardrum.
- **Inner ear:** Your inner ear contains sensory receptors that provide your hearing and balance. The hearing receptors are enclosed in the *cochlea,* a fluid-filled chamber, while the balance receptors are in the semicircular canals (refer to Figure 5-2).
- **Eustachian tube (ET):** Your Eustachian tube is an extension of the middle ear that connects to the nasopharynx. The ET, often the origin of ear infections, serves three important functions. It provides ventilation for your middle ear, helps equalize air pressure inside your ear (buffering the eardrum from the force of external air), and helps dissipate the energy of sound waves from your inner ear into your throat. And because it's closed most of the time, your ET serves as an important barrier to viruses, bacteria, irritants, and allergens that enter your middle ear.

  Similar to the function of your sinuses, cilia in the middle ear sweep debris-laden mucus from your middle ear through the ET into the back of your nasal cavity. The cilia prepare the mucus for drainage into your throat and eventually into your stomach. The ET briefly opens to allow the cilia to sweep mucus away when you swallow, yawn, sniff, or strain. In many children, however, the ET doesn't fully develop until age 6, causing the ET to ineffectively ventilate, clear, or protect the middle ear. Large numbers of young children get middle ear infections.

Acute otitis media (AOM)

Many people suffer from *acute otitis media* (an inflammation and infection of the middle ear and Eustachian tube) in early childhood. Symptoms are

- Earache — sometimes with intense stabbing pains — and fever. Occasionally, vomiting and diarrhea accompany this symptom.
- Possible hearing loss and occasional dizziness and ringing in the affected ear.
- With infants, high fever, irritability, and a tendency to pull on the affected ear.
- In some cases, discharge of infected fluid from the middle ear (if your eardrum has been perforated).

An AOM infection generally develops as a result of an allergic, bacterial, or viral ailment that inflames your nose, sinuses, middle ear, and Eustachian tube. Your ET may swell shut, trapping infected fluid, which then presses on your eardrum, causing the pain you associate with an earache. If you don't rectify this situation, infected fluids can eventually reach the membranes that cover your brain, leading to meningitis and even possibly death.

Because sinusitis and otitis media often coexist, doctors usually treat these conditions with the same medications. Treatment of AOM usually includes a course of antibiotics (available by prescription only) to rid your middle ear of infection. The antibiotic drugs that doctors commonly prescribe include

- Amoxicillin (Amoxil) or amoxicillin/potassium clavulanate (Augmentin)
- Clarithromycin (Biaxin) or azithromycin (Zithromax)

- Trimethoprim-sulfamethoxazole (Bactrim or Septra)
- A third-generation cephalosporin antibiotic, such as cefuroxime (Ceftin), cefpodoxime (Vantin), cefprozil (Cefzil), and cefixime (Suprax)

If you're allergic to penicillin, make sure your doctor knows. Some people who have penicillin allergies may also have adverse reactions to cephalosporin medications.

Otitis media with effusion (OME)

When you have otitis media with effusion (OME, also known as *serous otitis media*), your middle ear traps infected or sterile fluid. Common symptoms are

- Plugged-up ears (similar to the discomfort you may experience when descending in an airplane)
- Some hearing loss

Children with OME may not show obvious symptoms. However, if your child acts inattentive (other than the obvious times when children don't seem to hear you asking them to clean their room), doesn't seem to hear well (for example, he or she always wants the television volume turned up loud), and/or talks loudly, make sure your doctor examines your child's ears. Undetected or poorly treated OME can result in hearing loss, poor language development, learning disorders, and eventual behavioral problems.

OME treatments can also include nonprescription oral decongestants and nasal decongestant sprays as well as topical nasal corticosteroid sprays. (For more on these types of medicines, see Chapters 3 and 4.)

For children with chronic OME that lasts more than six to eight weeks, your pediatrician may refer your child to an ENT specialist for surgery. The most common OME treatment procedures are

- **Adenoidectomy:** If your child's Eustachian tube is chronically blocked and your child is more than 3 years old, your doctor may recommend removing your child's adenoids. (Removing the tonsils is no longer an effective or appropriate procedure for treatment of ear problems.)
- **Myringotomy:** The ENT surgeon makes a small incision in the eardrum that permits drainage of the trapped fluid. This procedure is helpful both for diagnostic purposes (to identify infecting organisms) and to relieve the severe pain, pressure, and fever associated with an acute middle ear infection.
- **Tympanostomy:** This procedure includes surgically inserting small plastic tubes (known as *pressure equalization* or *PE tubes*) in the eardrum to equalize air pressure in the ear and to allow drainage of fluid from the middle ear and Eustachian tube down to the nasopharynx. ENT surgeons usually perform tympanostomies with a general anesthetic and occasionally with local anesthetic (for older children or adults) as an outpatient procedure. In most cases, doctors recommend that PE tubes remain in place for 6 to 18 months or until they fall out. Children often don't notice the tubes after they've been in place for a while. Generally, children with tubes shouldn't go swimming. However, in some cases, an ENT surgeon may fit your child with earplugs, making water activities a possibility.

Diagnosing ear infections

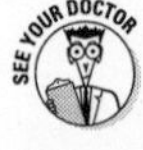

The first step in diagnosing suspected ear infections usually involves examining your middle ear. Your doctor usually uses an *otoscope* (a metal instrument you've probably seen before) to look for an obvious sign of infection. AOM often appears as a swollen, red, inflamed bulging of the tympanic membrane (eardrum) with poor or no movement. OME can appear as a pink or white, opaque, withdrawn tympanic membrane with poor or no movement.

Other diagnostic procedures for AOM and OME are

- **Audiometry:** This procedure evaluates the effect of chronic middle ear effusions on a person's hearing. Audiometry is especially important for children, because hearing loss can cause delayed speech and language development.
- **Tympanometry:** This procedure measures the eardrum's response at various pressure levels and helps to diagnose middle ear effusions and Eustachian tube dysfunction.

Taking preventive measures

As with sinusitis, one important step you can take to prevent ear infections, if you also have allergic rhinitis, is to effectively treat your allergies, which includes avoiding certain allergens and also using the appropriate medications, if necessary, to manage allergic rhinitis symptoms (see Chapters 3 and 4).

You also need to take the preventive measures that I describe in the "Complicating Your Allergies: Sinusitis" section of this chapter to keep your sinuses clear if you have an allergy attack or a cold or other upper respiratory infection.

Chapter 6

A Primer on Food Allergies

In This Chapter

- Categorizing adverse food reactions
- Investigating allergic and nonallergic food hypersensitivities
- Understanding how food intolerance differs from food hypersensitivity
- Getting medical attention for severe food reactions
- Preventing allergic food reactions

If the food you eat bites you back with fits of wheezing, outbreaks of eczema, gastric distress, or other symptoms (perhaps even including life-threatening bouts of anaphylactic shock), you're not alone. Adverse food reactions affect at least one in four Americans at some point in their lives. Food allergies can even trigger asthma symptoms that, in some cases, cause life-threatening respiratory symptoms in certain susceptible asthmatics.

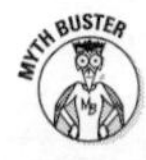

However, not all food ingredients that can cause adverse reactions are triggers of *food hypersensitivity* (the more precise term for *food allergy*). Even though 40 percent of Americans believe that their unfortunate gastronomical experiences result from allergies to certain foods, most cases involve various forms of food intolerance, food poisoning, and other types of nonallergic conditions.

Types of Adverse Food Reactions

Because the range of adverse food reactions can include a constellation of nasal, respiratory, skin, gastrointestinal, and oral symptoms, occurring separately or in combination, doctors usually classify these reactions according to the mechanisms that the reactions involve.

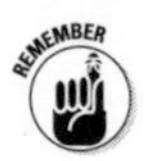

The following list summarizes the two main classifications of adverse food reactions:

- **Food hypersensitivity:** These reactions occur when your immune system responds to specific proteins in certain foods. The reactions can include allergic mechanisms involving IgE antibodies as well as nonallergic mechanisms.

  Allergic food hypersensitivities include gastrointestinal (GI) tract allergies, hives and other allergic skin reactions, and even *anaphylaxis* (a severe, abrupt reaction that affects many organs of the body simultaneously and can potentially be life-threatening).

  Nonallergic food hypersensitivities (sometimes referred to as *non-IgE food reactions*) include syndromes such as food-induced enterocolitis, colitis, and malabsorption, as well as celiac disease, dermatitis herpetiformis, and pulmonary hypersensitivity. I discuss these medical conditions in greater detail in "Nonallergic (Non-IgE) Food Hypersensitivities," later in this chapter.

- **Food intolerance:** These types of reactions result from nonallergic, nonimmunologic responses to offending substances in various foods. Forms of food intolerance include lactose intolerance, pharmacologic food reactions, metabolic food reactions, food additive reactions, food poisoning, and toxic reactions.

Although allergic reactions to food can be severe (and should be appropriately diagnosed and managed), the actual number of adults in the United States who suffer from true food hypersensitivities is close to 1 percent of the population. However, food allergies may affect as many as 6 percent of infants and children, with allergic reactions to peanuts topping the list of triggers of severe, even life-threatening respiratory symptoms in some children with asthma. According to one recent study of life-threatening asthma attacks, half of the children hospitalized in these cases had food hypersensitivities, especially to peanuts.

Allergic Food Hypersensitivities

In the case of *IgE-mediated food hypersensitivity,* commonly known as a *food allergy,* your immune system cooks up specific IgE antibodies against specific allergens. The level of exposure required for your immune system to be sensitized to a particular food varies, depending on the allergens involved. The major food allergens that have been identified are mostly proteins, often found in the following foods:

- Peanuts (the leading cause of severe allergic food reactions), soybeans, peas, lentils, beans and other legumes, and foods containing these products as ingredients. Because a wide variety of foods include peanuts and soybean products as ingredients, these legumes often act as hidden triggers of food allergies. See "Anaphylaxis and allergic food reactions," later in this chapter, for more on peanut issues. Likewise, you can find details on uncovering hidden allergenic ingredients in many common foods in "Avoiding Adverse Food Reactions," later in this chapter.

- Shellfish, such as shrimp, lobster, crab, clams, and oysters.
- Fish — both freshwater and saltwater.
- Tree nuts, including almonds, Brazil nuts, cashews, hazelnuts, and walnuts.
- Eggs, especially egg whites, which contain the predominant allergenic proteins, ovalbumin and ovomucoid. The yolk is less allergenic than the egg white.
- Cow's milk and products that contain milk protein fractions, such as *casein* (80 percent of the protein in cow's milk) and whey, which includes lactalbumin and lactoglobulin.
- Wheat, an important ingredient in bran, malt, wheat flour, graham flour, wheat germ, and wheat starch. Corn, rice, barley, oats, and other grains and cereals are less common food allergy triggers.

Of the preceding culprits, the products that trigger allergic food reactions in children most frequently are milk, eggs, peanuts, tree nuts, fish, soy, and wheat. In adults, the likeliest causes of allergic food reactions include fish, shellfish, peanuts, and tree nuts.

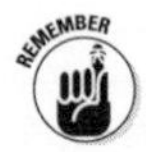

Although most children lose their sensitivity to milk and eggs by age 3, food allergies involving peanuts, fish, shellfish, and tree nuts can last a lifetime.

Other, less obvious sources of food allergens may possibly cause adverse reactions in a smaller number of susceptible individuals. These much less frequently

Hives and other food-related skin reactions

Allergic food hypersensitivities involving IgE antibodies can also trigger skin reactions in people whose atopic predisposition shows up through skin conditions. These conditions include

- ***Atopic dermatitis* (eczema):** Eggs, milk, peanuts, tree nuts, soybeans, and wheat can contribute to outbreaks in more than one-third of children affected by this skin condition.
- ***Urticaria* (hives):** These itchy welts can erupt from various types of reactions to many foods, including peanuts, tree nuts, milk, eggs, fish, shellfish, soybeans, and fruits, as well as food additives such as sodium benzoates, sulfites, and food dyes. Skin contact with raw meats, fish, vegetables, and fruit can also trigger hives. Allergic-food hypersensitivities are more likely to act as triggers of *rapid-onset urticaria* (a particularly quick and severe eruption of hives) in children than in adults. Food-related, exercise-induced anaphylaxis, which I discuss later in this chapter, can also trigger hives and angioedema.
- ***Angioedema:*** Also known as *deep swellings,* this condition results in deeper tissue inflammation and skin swelling and is more likely to produce painful and burning sensations rather than itching. Angioedema can erupt as a reaction to the same food allergens that trigger hives.

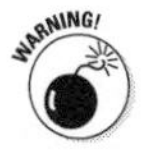

In severe cases of hives and angioedema, symptoms can also include swelling of the tongue, throat, airway, and difficulty swallowing, as well as fainting. If angioedema affects your face, the swelling may potentially lead to breathing difficulties. If you experience swelling of your airway, get emergency care immediately.

Anaphylaxis and allergic food reactions

The most extreme of all allergic food symptoms is *anaphylaxis*. This abrupt, systemic allergic reaction, often caused by the same foods that trigger hives and angioedema, affects several organs simultaneously and can quickly turn life-threatening. In recent years, the incidence of this severe and sometimes fatal reaction has been rising at an alarming rate among asthmatics, with most of these episodes due to accidental ingestion of peanuts, tree nuts, or seafood.

What is particularly disturbing is the fact that so many of these known high-risk patients are aware of their diagnosis but still don't carry appropriate emergency medication, such as an epinephrine kit, when they experience their anaphylactic reaction or don't receive immediate, potentially life-saving emergency care in time.

If you're an asthma patient or susceptible to food allergy–related anaphylactic reactions, keep emergency medication with you at all times. Wear a MedicAlert bracelet, especially children in school.

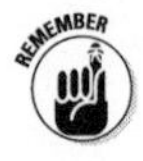

Generalized urticaria (widespread hives occurring simultaneously over much of your body surface area) can often be the initial symptom of impending anaphylaxis and can result in a sudden swelling *(angioedema)* of the lips, eyelids, tongue, and windpipe *(laryngeal edema)* as well as wheezing and dizziness. This particularly dangerous reaction can quickly progress to anaphylaxis, leading to shock, hypotension, *arrhythmia* (irregular heartbeat), and even cardiorespiratory arrest. In rare cases, this type of reaction can be fatal.

Common triggers of total body hives include

- Foods such as peanuts and shellfish (in people who have extreme hypersensitivities to these foods)
- Severe allergic reactions to medications such as penicillin and related compounds
- Generalized hypersensitivity to latex
- Extreme sensitivities to insect stings, including those of honeybees, yellow jackets, wasps, hornets, and fire ants

Food-dependent, exercise-induced anaphylaxis, a variant of exercise-induced anaphylaxis, can occur when you exercise within three to four hours after eating a particular food. Two forms of this condition exist.

- You may develop anaphylaxis if you ingest particular foods, especially celery, shellfish, wheat, fruit, milk, or fish, prior to exercise. If you experience this reaction and can identify the specific foods that trigger episodes, your doctor may advise allergy skin testing (see Chapter 2) to confirm your sensitivity to the suspected foods.
- You may develop anaphylaxis while exercising, regardless of the type of food you've consumed.

As a parent of a peanut-allergic child, you need to pay close attention to products that may contain peanuts, because they can potentially cause life-threatening anaphylactic reactions in children (as well as adults) who are extremely allergic to this food.

Keep the following important points in mind about peanuts and children:

- Many foods contain peanuts as a not-so-obvious added ingredient. Therefore, examine all food labels for peanut ingredients and carefully select menu items when dining out with a child who is allergic to peanuts. (See "Avoiding Adverse Food Reactions," later in this chapter, for more information on foods that contain peanuts.) You may want to pack your child's lunch to reduce the risk of your child unknowingly consuming foods with minute traces of peanuts in school lunches.

- Because many foods include peanuts as ingredients, instruct your young child not only to avoid peanuts but also never to accept foods — particularly snacks and candy bars — from others, especially playmates and young siblings.
- Because the peanut food allergy issue has received widespread media attention, some airlines are introducing peanut-free flights. If your child suffers from food allergies of any kind, however, ask questions about the food on your flight, even if the airline claims that no peanuts or peanut ingredients are in the snacks or meals.
- A child who has a peanut hypersensitivity should wear a MedicAlert bracelet, especially at school. Also, ask your family doctor about supplying your child's school with an emergency epinephrine kit. Make sure school personnel know how and when to administer this medication.

If you're prone to anaphylaxis, carry injectable epinephrine with you at all times and receive emergency care as soon as possible after an attack occurs. Make sure you have an emergency plan in place that includes the following items:

- Medications your doctor has prescribed for you in the event of an anaphylactic reaction
- A list of your symptoms
- A written treatment plan prepared by your physician
- Your physician's name and contact information

If you're treated for anaphylaxis, don't be surprised if you continue to be observed in the emergency room for several hours after responding to initial rescue therapy. Unfortunately, in a few cases, patients who have responded well to initial anaphylaxis treatment have been immediately discharged from the emergency room but, within a few hours, experienced a severe late-phase, or second reaction, known as *biphasic anaphylaxis.*

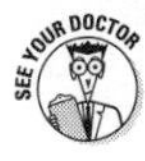

Ask your doctor whether an emergency epinephrine kit, such as an EpiPen (or EpiPen Jr. for children under 66 pounds), with an injectable dose of epinephrine, is advisable for you or your child. Parents and caregivers of children under 30 pounds (about 14 kilograms), who are too small for the dose of a preloaded EpiPen Jr., should be taught how to properly administer the correct dose of epinephrine by syringe to their infant or young child. Wear a MedicAlert bracelet or necklace in case you're unable to speak during a reaction.

Food hypersensitivity is a leading cause of anaphylaxis. Current estimates are that as many as 125 people in the United States die each year from food-induced anaphylactic reactions. As you may expect, the most effective long-term method for preventing food-induced anaphylactic reactions is to avoid eating foods that trigger the reaction. I provide more details on avoiding food allergens and establishing a safe diet in "Avoiding Adverse Food Reactions," later in this chapter.

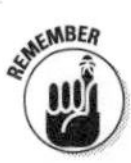

If your child suffers from food-induced anaphylaxis, notify babysitters, relatives, other children's parents, daycare workers, teachers, and other school personnel of your child's sensitivities.

Nonallergic (Non-IgE) Food Hypersensitivities

You can also have food hypersensitivity from immune system reactions that don't involve the production of IgE antibodies. The most significant nonallergic food reactions include the following:

- **Food-induced enterocolitis syndrome:** This condition primarily occurs in infants between 1 and 3 months of age. Characteristic symptoms include prolonged vomiting and diarrhea, often resulting in dehydration. Triggers are usually the proteins in formulas that contain cow's milk or soy substitutes. Occasionally, breastfed infants may also suffer from this syndrome, presumably as the result of a protein ingested by the mother and transferred to the infant in maternal milk. Similar symptoms can occur in older children and adults in response to eggs, rice, wheat, and peanuts. However, most children outgrow this type of hypersensitivity by their third birthday.
- **Food-induced colitis:** Cow's milk and soy protein hypersensitivity have been implicated in this disorder, which can occur in the first few months of life and is usually diagnosed through the presence of blood in the stools, seen either by the naked eye or hidden *(occult),* of children who otherwise appear healthy. This condition often diminishes after 6 months to 2 years if children avoid the implicated food allergens. Feeding a hypoallergenic formula to your baby may help overcome food-induced colitis.
- **Malabsorption syndrome:** This condition involves hypersensitivities to proteins in foods such as cow's milk, soy, wheat and other cereal grains, and eggs. Symptoms include diarrhea, vomiting, and weight loss or failure to gain weight.

- **Celiac disease:** This condition is a more serious form of malabsorption syndrome, and it can cause intestinal inflammation. Symptoms range from diarrhea and abdominal cramping to anemia and osteoporosis. Celiac disease only seems to occur in people who inherit an atopic predisposition. Affected individuals develop a hypersensitivity to a component of gluten called *gliadin,* which you find in wheat, oats, rye, and barley. If you suffer from this syndrome, however, you're not necessarily doomed to a life without pasta and pancakes. Resourceful sufferers of celiac disease have come up with many gluten-free products, ranging from beer to pretzels.
- **Dermatitis herpetiformis:** This condition is a non-IgE-mediated food hypersensitivity to gluten that produces skin eruptions in addition to causing intestinal inflammation. The typical symptom includes a chronic, itchy rash that appears primarily on the elbows, knees, and buttocks, although the disease can affect other areas as well.
- **Pulmonary hypersensitivity:** This rare condition, induced by cow's milk, primarily affects young children. Characteristic symptoms include a chronic cough, wheezing, and severe anemia. Removing the offending dairy products from the diet can substantially alleviate symptoms.

Differences between Food Allergy and Food Intolerance

As I explain earlier in this chapter, many adverse food reactions don't involve an immune system response. These types of direct, nonimmunologic reactions are considered signs and symptoms of food intolerance and include the conditions in the following sections.

Lactose intolerance

If you're lactose intolerant, odds are your body doesn't produce sufficient amounts of the lactase enzyme in order for you to properly digest cow's milk. If you drink milk or consume foods with high milk content, you may experience stomach cramps, bloating, nausea, gas, and diarrhea.

Avoiding cow's milk and cow's milk products or adding the lactase enzyme to those foods are the standard ways of managing lactose intolerance. In contrast with the cow's-milk allergy (which I mention earlier in "Allergic Food Hypersensitivities"), you may be able to consume small quantities of cow's milk without suffering an adverse reaction.

Metabolic food reactions

In some cases, eating average or normal amounts of particular foods (especially fatty foods) may disrupt your digestive system. These disruptions, called *metabolic food reactions,* may be caused by

- Medications (for example, antibiotics) you're taking for illnesses
- A disease or condition (such as a gastrointestinal virus) that may affect your digestive system
- Malnutrition (for example, due to vitamin or enzyme deficiency)

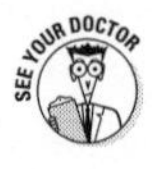

Always remember to ask your doctor if any medication you're taking might disrupt your digestive system.

Pharmacologic food reactions

More serious forms of metabolic food reactions can result if you combine certain foods and drugs that don't mix well. Beware of the following potentially dangerous combinations:

- Grapefruit juice, which is usually harmless, sometimes causes harmful interactions when taken with calcium channel blockers, such as Procardia. If you have a heart condition, ask your doctor about possible interactions between grapefruit juice and any over-the-counter (OTC) or prescription antihistamines you may take.
- If you take blood-thinning drugs such as Coumadin, check with your doctor before eating foods rich in vitamin K like broccoli, spinach, and turnip greens, because they can reduce the medications' effectiveness.
- A harmful potassium buildup can occur if you overindulge on bananas while taking ACE inhibitors, such as Capoten and Vasotec.
- Avoid foods high in tyramine, such as cheese and sausage, if you take MAO inhibitors, because the combination can cause a potentially fatal rise in blood pressure. Tyramine may also aggravate or trigger migraine headaches.
- The caffeine in coffee, tea, and colas can interact badly with ulcer medications such as Tagamet, Zantac, and Pepcid AC. If your doctor prescribes theophylline for your asthma, reduce your caffeine intake, because caffeine can worsen side effects, such as GI irritation, headache, jitteriness, and sleeplessness.

Food additive reactions

Doctors associate many types of food additives with adverse food reactions. The most frequently implicated food additives are

- **Monosodium glutamate (MSG):** When consumed in large quantities, this flavor enhancer reportedly causes burning sensations, facial pressure, chest pain, headache, and, in rare cases, severe asthma symptoms. Although many sufferers associate these types of reactions with eating Chinese or other types of Asian foods, no conclusive studies have determined a clear link between consuming MSG and adverse food reactions. In any event, with the recent increase of MSG-free restaurants in many parts of the United States, you should have no trouble finding a place to chow down on chow mein without suffering ill effects.
- **Tartrazine (yellow dye No. 5):** This and other food dyes can aggravate chronic hives and may actually be an ingredient in the very same children's syrups used to treat allergic symptoms such as hives — another good reason to always check medication labels.
- **Sulfites:** Commonly found in processed foods and almost always in wines, sulfites can produce respiratory difficulties. In some cases, sulfites can also trigger potentially life-threatening airway constriction and asthma symptoms in some individuals (see the sidebar "Additives and allergies," earlier in this chapter).

Food poisoning

Food poisoning can result from bacterial contamination of improperly prepared or handled foods, especially meats or salads. You've probably heard of bacterial bad guys such as salmonella,

E. coli, listeria, and staphylococcus enterotoxin. These bacteria are the usual suspects in outbreaks of food poisoning. Food poisoning symptoms typically include nausea, vomiting, and diarrhea and can often mimic the flu. In rare cases, food-poisoning reactions can be fatal if not treated in time.

Researchers believe that many cases of illness mistakenly diagnosed as the 24-hour flu bug are actually the result of ingesting tainted foods. A particular reaction from spoiled fish, known as *scombroidosis,* can mimic food allergy due to the release of histamine-like chemicals. Itching, hives, and even shortness of breath can occur, depending on the amount of spoiled fish a person has eaten.

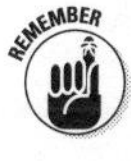

If many people develop similar symptoms after eating the same meal (the potato salad that sat in the sun all afternoon at the family picnic, for example), food poisoning is the likely cause of all those urgent trips to the restroom.

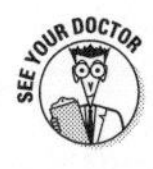

If you experience severe gastric distress that seems related to food poisoning, make sure you drink enough liquid to avoid dehydration, which is one of the most serious adverse effects. If your condition doesn't improve within 24 hours, seek medical attention.

Diagnosing Adverse Food Reactions

In order to diagnose your adverse food reactions, your physician should take a detailed medical history and conduct a physical examination. Your doctor may also ask you about the specific details of your reactions to figure out what may be causing your reactions.

Keeping a food diary

A detailed food diary, in which you record everything you consume (even those midnight snacks) and describe your reactions, can help your doctor diagnose your condition.

A well-kept food diary can assist you in telling your doctor about the following items:

- The timing of your reactions. For example, do they occur immediately after you've consumed a food or liquid and, if not, how long afterward?
- The amount of food that seems to trigger a reaction.
- Where and how the food was prepared.
- The duration and severity of your symptoms.
- Any activities, especially exercise, associated with your reactions.

Considering atopic causes

As part of the physical examination, your doctor should also look for signs of atopic diseases, including

- Dry, scaly skin, which can indicate eczema
- Dark circles under your eyes, which may indicate hay fever
- Wheezing and coughing, which can signal asthma symptoms

Eliminating possible food culprits

In some cases, your doctor may advise an *elimination diet* for you as a way of confirming what triggers your adverse reactions. This process involves eliminating suspected foods from your diet, one at a time, under your doctor's supervision. If your symptoms significantly improve, your doctor may then gradually reintroduce the likeliest food suspect to determine whether it's the source of your woes.

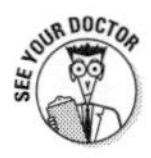

Only undertake an elimination diet under your physician's direction. You don't want to deprive yourself of foods that may not cause your symptoms and are vital for your overall health. Your doctor may also advise an elimination diet in order to prepare you for an oral food challenge, which I describe in the following section.

Testing for food allergens

If your doctor can't readily identify the cause of your reactions, he or she may also recommend confirming a suspected food allergen with the following allergy tests.

Skin testing involves using specific food extracts to evaluate your sensitivity to suspected allergens. Only a qualified specialist, such as an allergist, should perform skin testing. Skin testing for food allergens isn't always recommended.

In some cases, your doctor may not advise skin testing, because a positive reaction may involve unacceptable risks of inducing anaphylactic shock, particularly if you're highly sensitized to certain foods, such as peanuts.

In general, prick-puncture tests are the only skin tests that your doctor needs to administer when attempting to identify suspected food allergens. (See Chapter 2 for more about prick-puncture tests.)

Oral food challenges involve actually ingesting — under medical supervision — minute quantities of food that contain suspected allergens.

To ensure the most accurate diagnosis, your doctor should administer an oral food challenge while you're symptom-free, usually as a result of a food elimination diet. Depending on the severity of your adverse food reactions and the type of food allergen that your physician suspects as the cause, your doctor may choose to administer one or more of the following types of oral food challenges:

- **Open challenge:** In this type of test, your doctor informs you of what type of food you're ingesting.
- **Single-blind challenge:** With this test, your doctor doesn't inform you of what you're eating. However, your doctor or the clinician administering the test knows the ingredients.
- **Double-blind, placebo-controlled oral food challenge (DBPCOFC):** This elaborate procedure is the gold standard for identifying food allergens. Neither you nor your doctor (nor the clinician who administers the test) knows the contents of the test. A third party, such as a nurse or a lab technician, prepares the opaque capsule for testing. In most cases, your doctor schedules a DBPCOFC so you can fast for a prescribed amount of time beforehand. You also need to stop taking antihistamines (based on your doctor's advice) prior to the challenge, because these drugs can interfere with the accuracy. The initial dose of the suspected food in this test is usually half of the minimum quantity that your doctor estimates as the trigger for your reaction. After the test, the technician identifies the capsule's contents to help your doctor make the proper diagnosis.

  Take this challenge only in a facility equipped to treat potentially severe reactions. If your history of adverse food reactions is life-threatening, your doctor will most likely advise you that an oral food challenge is too risky.

Your doctor may recommend *radioallergensorbent testing,* a type of blood test that measures levels of food-specific IgE antibodies in your blood, if skin testing or oral food challenges seem too risky. Most allergists rarely use RAST, because it isn't as accurate as skin testing and may result in an incomplete profile of your allergies. For more information on this test, see Chapter 2.

Avoiding Adverse Food Reactions

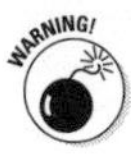

After your doctor determines the source of your adverse food reactions, the most effective long-term approach to managing your condition and preventing further reactions is strict avoidance of the implicated food. Avoidance may seem like an obvious solution. However, you may need to become an expert at reading ingredient listings when you buy groceries. In some cases, food allergens and other types of precipitants may hide under arcane names in food labels. Hidden ingredients in many processed and packaged foods may also be sources of problematic allergens.

For updates and information on food allergens and related issues and to find out how to decipher ingredients listed on food labels, contact the Food Allergy & Anaphylaxis Network at 800-929-4040 or visit the organization's Web site at `www.foodallergy.org`.

Make sure that your family, friends, and colleagues all understand what causes your adverse food reactions. You can then minimize the chances of erupting in hives at your Thanksgiving meal or during that crucial dinner with your boss and the company's new clients.

If you have a life-threatening food allergy, you may need to avoid certain restaurants. In many cases, food servers don't have enough information about the ingredients in the establishment's menu to guarantee you an allergen-free meal, although some restaurants actually do offer dishes without common food allergens. However, double-check all the ingredients in the menu item with the chef or restaurant manager. In particular, inquire whether the restaurant prepares allergen-free meals using surfaces, cookware, fryers, and utensils that are separated from the other items in the kitchen.

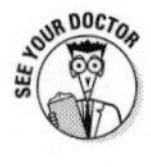

If effective management of your adverse food reactions involves excluding common food groups from your diet for long periods, consider professional dietary advice in order to prevent nutritional deficiency or malnutrition.

Chapter 7

Ten Tips for Traveling with Allergies and Asthma

In This Chapter

- Making sensible travel plans
- Taking medications and other essentials with you
- Dealing with problems on the road
- Attending to children while traveling

If only airlines could lose your allergies and asthma the way they sometimes lose your baggage. Imagine if you could leave your wheezing instead of your heart in San Francisco. And wouldn't waking up in the city that never sleeps because the Big Apple stirs you to the very core — instead of allergies or asthma interrupting a good night's rest — be nice?

Of course, getting away from allergies and asthma isn't that easy. Think of asthma and often-related conditions, such as *allergic rhinitis* (hay fever), as constant companions. Wherever you may roam, these conditions will be along for the ride. Knowing how to control the symptoms of these ailments is vital to ensuring that no matter what else may go wrong during your travel, your condition won't complicate or ruin your plans.

Planning a Safe, Healthy Trip

A key element in proper travel planning is avoiding places where you know pollens, dander, tobacco smoke, or other allergens and irritants may be prevalent and could, depending on your specific sensitivities, trigger your respiratory and/or allergy symptoms. Here are general guidelines for preventing problems frequently associated with dander, food allergens, and ragweed while away from home:

- **Dander:** Beware of visiting or staying in homes with cats, dogs, and other animals, including rabbits, birds, and gerbils and other domesticated rodents. Even if the animal lover removes the pet from the area, you can still suffer an adverse reaction because of the residual dander and/or hair in the room. Horseback riding also may not be advisable. Before you saddle up for a dude ranch out West, make sure you can control any symptoms that Trigger's horsehair may just trigger. Consult your doctor about preventive medications.
- **Food allergens:** The foods that trigger allergic reactions most frequently in adults with food hypersensitivities include fish, shellfish, peanuts, and tree nuts. For children, the most common triggers are milk, eggs, peanuts, tree nuts, fish, soy, and wheat (see Chapter 6). Because of the swiftness and severity with which a food allergy reaction can strike (especially with peanuts), be especially vigilant in avoiding these triggers when traveling. In particular, if you or your child is sensitive to peanuts and you're planning to

travel where these seemingly harmless legumes are a regular part of local cuisine (many parts of East Asia, for example), ask your doctor about additional precautions you can take. Although you can clearly identify peanuts in many dishes, they may be a hidden part of the cooking process itself in many cases (for example, foods cooked alongside dishes prepared with peanut products). When in doubt, avoid local fare in these parts of the world rather than risk reactions such as an asthma attack, hives, or, worse yet, a potentially life-threatening case of anaphylaxis (see Chapter 6).

- **Ragweed:** Avoiding travel to the eastern half of the United States and Canada from mid-August through October is probably advisable (assuming you don't already live there) if you're sensitized to ragweed pollen. If you must travel to those areas during ragweed season, ask your physician about preventive medications that you can take to keep your symptoms under control. Also, the National Allergy Bureau (NAB) of the American Academy of Allergy, Asthma, and Immunology (AAAAI) has seasonal allergen maps that chart the prevalence of allergenic pollens as well as several other allergens around the country throughout the year. Check out the NAB Web site at `www.aaaai.org/nab` or call 414-272-6071.

Adjusting Treatment for Travel

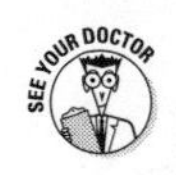

Prevention is the key to a safe and trouble-free trip, which usually means consulting your physician ahead of time to evaluate your allergy and asthma management and to make any advisable adjustments based on where and when you're going and what you'll be doing while traveling.

You may need to adjust your medication because of increased exposures to triggers. In addition, remember that changes in time zones may affect the dosage schedule of some medications you're taking (for any ailment, not just asthma or allergies).

You also need to make sure that you'll be able to stick with the program that your physician advises. If possible, get a letter from your doctor summarizing your medical history as well as the treatments and medications you're currently taking. If you're at risk of acute asthma or allergy attacks, ask your physician about wearing a MedicAlert bracelet on your wrist or pendant around your neck.

Taking Medications and Other Essentials

Have all your necessary medical supplies, devices, and prescriptions with you when traveling. If flying (or riding on a train or bus), keep these items in your carry-on bag. After you arrive at your destination, keep your essentials with you instead of leaving them in your hotel room (or other accommodation) when you're out and about. If you need to leave your medications in the room (for example, while using hotel recreational facilities), make sure you store these products in a safe and secure location, such as the room safe or in a locked suitcase, instead of leaving them out on the bathroom countertop.

Keep medications in their original containers and never mix pills of different types into one receptacle. By keeping them in their original containers, you'll have the proper dosage information readily available, which is especially important if someone else needs to administer your medication to you. Also, if you're traveling internationally, customs officials are generally less suspicious of pills and capsules in their original containers.

Getting Medications and Medical Help Abroad

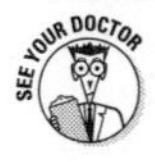

Ask your doctor about special medical considerations for specific countries and areas. Some countries require that you take certain vaccine shots before your visit. As for medications, don't assume that every place you visit has pharmacies stocked with the supplies you need. Write down both the brand names of your medications and their generic names. In a pinch, having both names available may allow a local pharmacist to find what you need.

When planning your trip, you may want to obtain a booklet that lists qualified, English-speaking physicians in just about every country of the world. The International Association for Medical Assistance to Travelers (IAMAT), a voluntary organization based in Canada, offers this booklet. You can contact them in the United States at 716-754-4883 or via their Web site at www.iamat.org for further information.

Also, if you're a U.S. citizen, the U.S. State Department's American Citizens Services can provide help in case of an emergency. Call the State Department's Hotline for American Travelers, 202-647-5225, or check the State Department's Web site, www.state.gov, before your departure to receive information on contacting U.S. embassies and consulates for assistance with medical matters.

Flying with Allergens and Irritants

Studies show that airplane passenger cabins are some of the worst indoor dust mite and animal dander sites. Because airliners are tightly sealed environments that often lack adequate air filtering or cleaning, they often concentrate sky-high quantities of allergens and irritants that hundreds, even thousands, of passengers constantly track in with them.

Many airplane seats house thriving colonies of dust mites and their allergenic waste products. In addition, although all U.S., Canadian, and many European flights ban smoking anywhere on the aircraft (and in most parts of airport terminals), some international flights still allow smoking.

If exposure to tobacco smoke triggers symptoms, find out as much as possible about an air carrier's smoking policies. If your travel includes flying an airline that permits smoking, try to get seating as far away from the smoking section as possible.

Take my advice when you're planning air travel:

- **Pack your medications in a carry-on bag so they're immediately available in the event of a serious asthma episode and/or allergic reaction and in case the airline loses your luggage.** (You want to avoid finding yourself in strange territory without your medications.)
- **Stay hydrated during your flight.** Avoid alcohol and drink plenty of water. Not only does drinking water help minimize potential allergy and

asthma problems, but it also can put a dent in whatever jet lag you may otherwise develop.

- **If you have the opportunity/financial ability, consider upgrading to first or business class.** If available, the leather seats may be less likely to harbor allergy triggers, and, at the least, you'll give yourself more breathing (and leg) room.

Considering Allergy Shots and Travel

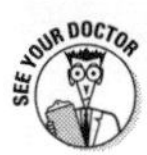

When you're traveling, I usually recommend transferring your immunotherapy (allergy shots) program to another location only if you'll be gone at least a month or more (if you're a snowbird from the North wintering in southern California or southern Florida, for example). If you'll be gone for a month or more, ask your physician for a referral to a doctor in the area where you'll be staying and have that physician administer your shots in a medical facility.

Although practices vary in different areas of the United States and the world, don't give yourself allergy shots. The risk, although low, of a bad reaction or even anaphylactic shock means you need qualified medical personnel around you, just in case (see Chapter 2).

When visiting the physician in the new location, bring your allergy serum (vaccine) vials in a refrigerated or ice-insulated pack and have clear written instructions from your doctor regarding your dose.

Reducing Trigger Exposures in Hotels and Motels

Tobacco smoke and its lingering traces can cause problems, especially outside the United States or Canada, where hotels and other accommodations are less likely to restrict smoking. Wherever you stay, reserve a room on a smoke-free floor. Likewise, if feathers pose a potential allergy problem for you, bring your own pillow and pillowcase.

Inspect the room before you occupy it, looking for signs of animal hair, dirty air vents, dust, or mold. If you find evidence suggesting that staying in the room will lead to breathing problems, ask for another room that appears safer and more comfortable. In some cases, your doctor may advise bringing along a portable HEPA air filter system. Check to see if your hotel offers allergy-free rooms, which may even come with HEPA filters and allergy covers on the mattresses.

Avoiding Food Allergies during Your Trip

In your travels, you may come into contact with foods to which you have an allergy (not just an intolerance — see Chapter 6). In some cases, the menu in a given restaurant, hotel, or cafe reveals all you need to know about potentially problematic ingredients. But more often than not, you need to ask a lot of questions about the cuisine and how it's prepared. Don't be rude but definitely don't be shy.

As I explain in Chapter 6, you may need to do more than simply determine that a particular dish doesn't contain foods to which you're allergic. For example, in many restaurants, various dishes are all prepared on the same grill. If you're allergic to shellfish, for example, make sure that the cooking surface and utensils used to prepare your food haven't also been previously used to prepare shellfish. If they have, allergens from the shellfish may end up in your meal, potentially causing a distressful dining experience.

If your food hypersensitivities put you at risk for anaphylaxis, wear a MedicAlert pendant or bracelet. Also ask your doctor about prescribing an epinephrine kit, such as an EpiPen (see Chapter 6), and be sure to carry the kit with you.

Finding Help in Case of Emergencies

Although the local hospital probably isn't at the top of your sightseeing list, find out the location of the nearest medical facility equipped to treat you in case of a serious adverse allergic reaction or severe asthma episode. Knowing where the closest help is available can help ensure that you get effective treatment if you experience a life-threatening reaction.

Depending on your destination, you can easily obtain local hospital locations from the organizations that I list earlier in "Getting Medications and Medical Help Abroad" or from your doctor or travel agent. In some cases, you may need to do more homework, but your health and safety are worth the effort.

Traveling with Children Who Have Allergies or Asthma

When traveling with a child who has allergies or asthma, many of the same considerations that adults must contend with also apply:

- **Pack two containers of all medications and make sure that you've labeled them properly.** Keep one container as a carry-on with you and keep the other in a purse, backpack, or briefcase.
- **Obtain a MedicAlert bracelet or necklace for your child to wear.** If you're not around, emergency medical personnel will immediately know what to do about your child's condition.
- **Show your child how to pack his or her asthma and/or allergy medications properly.** In addition to preparing your child for trips that he or she may take without you, this lesson can also help your youngster find out more about managing his or her condition appropriately.
- **Take at least two epinephrine kits (such as an EpiPen or EpiPen Jr. for children under 66 pounds) if your child is at risk for anaphylaxis to ensure that you'll always have one at hand.** Make sure that you and/or your child (depending on the youngster's age) know how to use the kit. You should receive instructions on the proper use of the injector in your doctor's office instead of waiting for a potential emergency to figure it out.
- **Ask questions about meals.** If your child has peanut allergies, be especially vigilant on airplanes (particularly with the contents of those appealingly packaged snack bags), where peanuts can be as common as delayed flights.

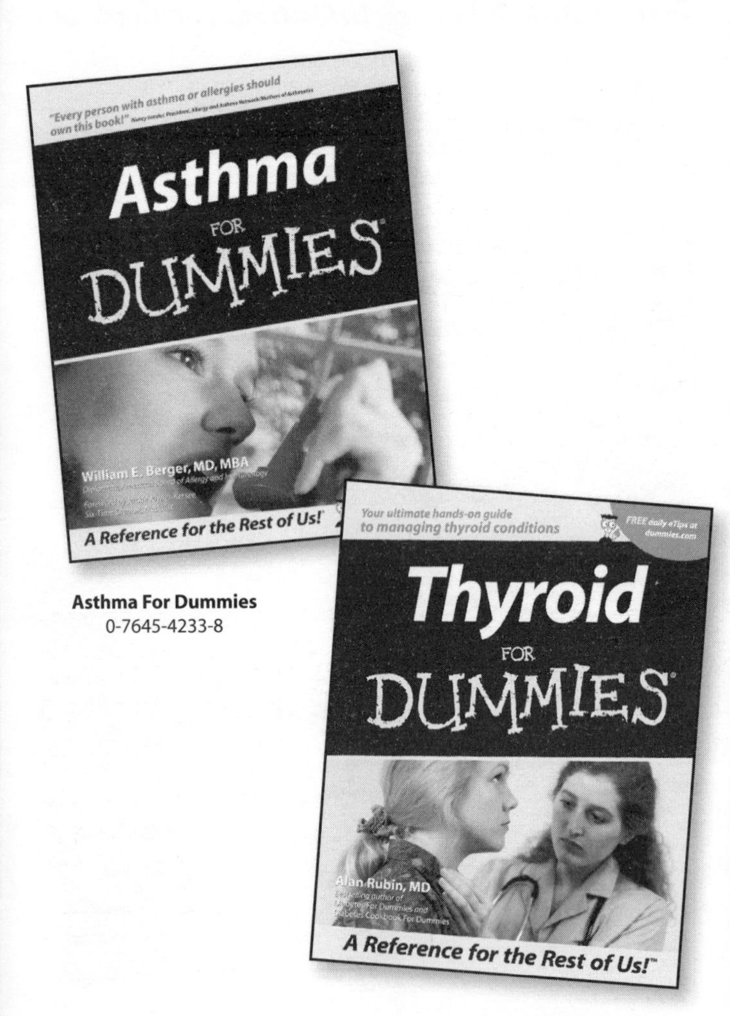

Asthma For Dummies
0-7645-4233-8

Thyroid For Dummies
0-7645-5385-2

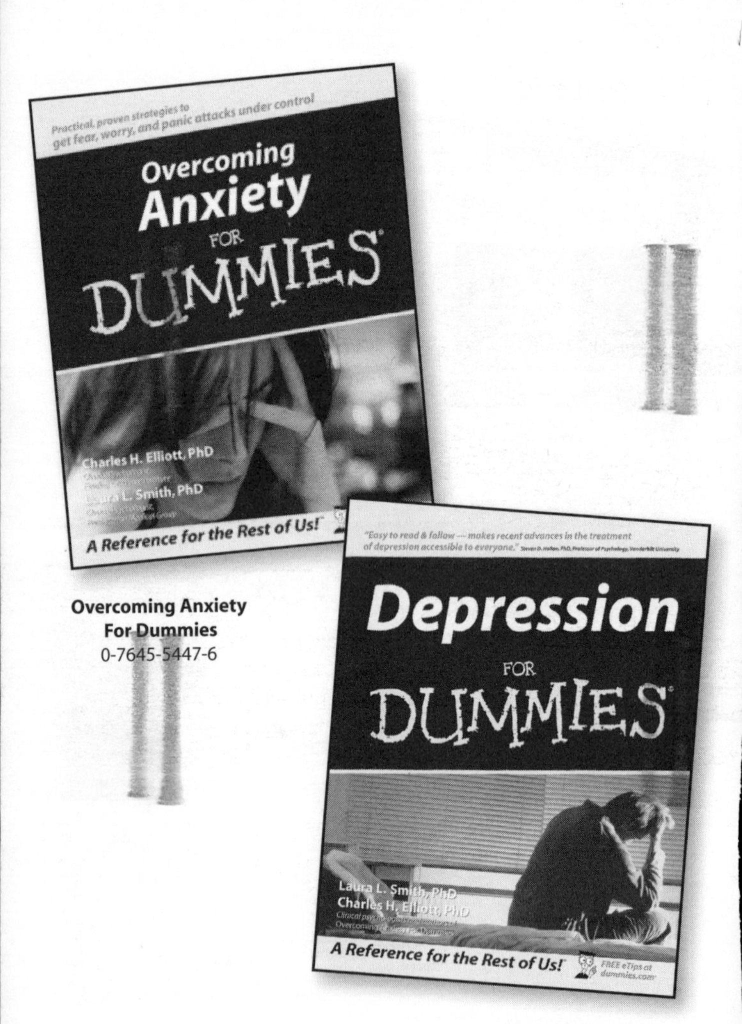

Overcoming Anxiety For Dummies
0-7645-5447-6

Depression For Dummies
0-7645-3900-0

After you've read the Pocket Edition, look for the original Dummies book on the topic. The handy Contents at a Glance below highlights the information you'll get when you purchase a copy of *Asthma For Dummies* – available wherever books are sold, or visit dummies.com.

Contents at a Glance

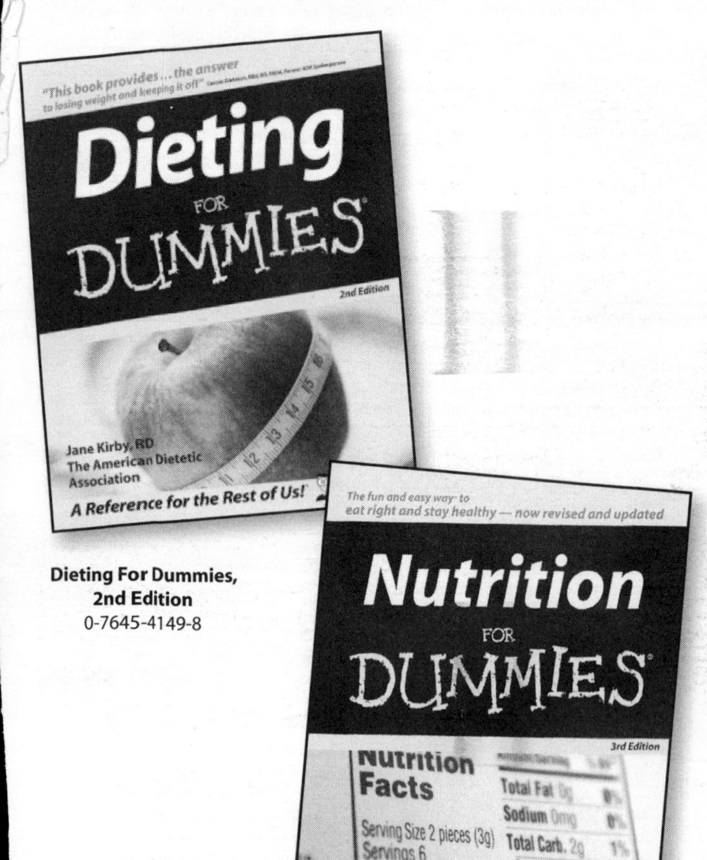

Dieting For Dummies,
2nd Edition
0-7645-4149-8

Nutrition For Dummies,
3rd Edition
0-7645-4082-3